The Grown-Up Girl's Guide to STYLE

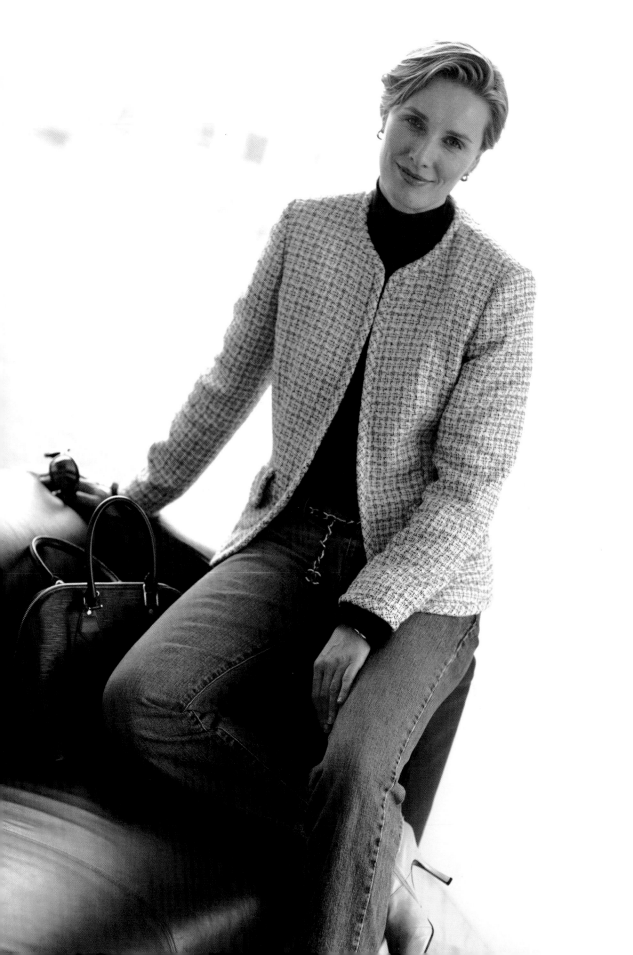

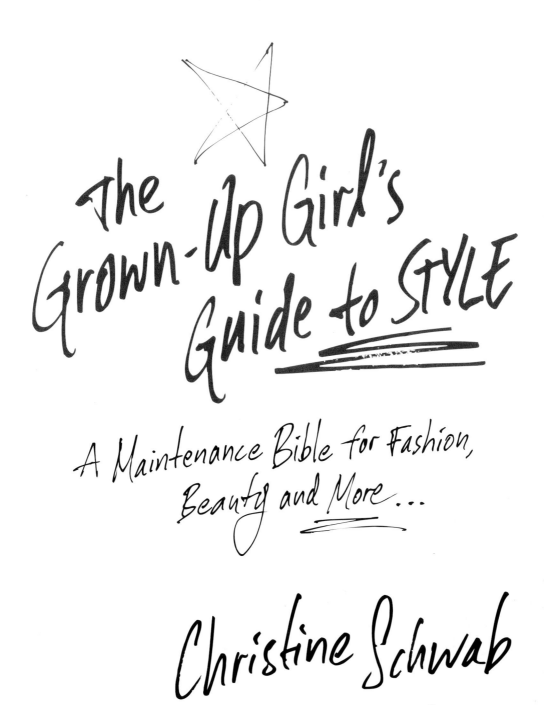

The Grown-Up Girl's Guide to STYLE

A Maintenance Bible for Fashion, Beauty and More...

Christine Schwab

REGAN

An Imprint of HarperCollinsPublishers

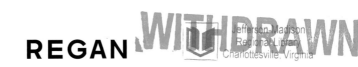

All photographs by Michael Donnelly, except for the following:

Pages 75, 80 (left), 146, and 204 by Luigi Ciuffetelli; page 4 by Tim Whitby/WireImage.com; page 5 by Kevin Winter/Getty Images; page 19 by Brenda Smialowski/Getty Images; page 23 (left) by George Chin/WireImage.com; page 23 (middle) by Steve Eichner/Photo Web/WireImage.com; page 23 (right) by Jeffrey Mayer/WireImage.com; page 26 (left) by Cochran/WireImage.com; page 26 (right) by Thos Robinson/Getty Images; page 27 by James Devaney/WireImage.com; page 34 by Vince Bucci/Getty Images; pages 39 and 111 by Steve Granitz/WireImage.com; page 65 by Carlo Allegri/Getty Images; page 77 (left) by Dimitros Kambouris/WireImage.com; page 83 (left) by Paul Hawthorne/Getty Images; pages 83 (right), 100, 126, and 136 by Kevin Mazur/WireImage.com; pages 77 (right) and 86 (left) by Gregory Pace/FilmMagic; pages 84, 86 (right), and 144 by Vera Anderson/WireImage.com; pages 90 (left) and 114 by Jean-Paul Aussenard/WireImage.com; page 123 (left) by Nuje Narskabd; page 123 (right) by Djamilla Rosa Cochran/WireImage.com; page 115 by Theo Wargo/WireImage.com; pages 133 and 158 by Kevin Parry/WireImage.com; pages 36, 37, 44, 71, 119, 120, 142, 180, 184, 186, and 187 from the author's personal collection; pages 6, 21, 22, 24, 29–32, 38, 39 (top), 40–43, 45, 52, 58, 59, 62, 63, 68, 69, 71 (top), 92, 93, 101–103, 108, 110, 124, 125, 127, 132, 171, 179, 193, 194, 199, 202, and 208 by Christine Schwab.

The advice contained herein is for informational purposes only. Please consult your medical professional before beginning any diet or exercise program. The author and publisher disclaim any liability for any damage resulting from the use of the information contained in this book.

HarperCollins books may be purchased for educational, business, or sales promotional use. For information please write: Special Markets Department, HarperCollins Publishers Inc., 10 East 53rd Street, New York, NY 10022.

For editorial inquiries, please contact Regan, 10100 Santa Monica Blvd., 10th floor, Los Angeles, CA 90067.

FIRST EDITION

Designed by Richard Ljoenes / Kris Tobiassen

Printed on acid-free paper

Library of Congress Cataloging-in-Publication Data

Schwab, Christine.
   The grown-up girl's guide to style : the maintenance bible for fashion, beauty, and more— / Christine Schwab.—1st ed.
      p. cm.
   ISBN-13: 978-0-06-078458-4 (alk. paper)
   ISBN-10: 0-06-078458-X (alk. paper)
   1. Beauty, Personal. 2. Middle-aged women—Clothing. 3. Women's clothing. 4. Fashion. I. Title.

   GT499.S38 2006
   646.7—dc22   2005057933

06 07 08 09 10 WBC/QUT 10 9 8 7 6 5 4 3 2 1

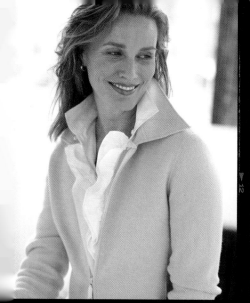
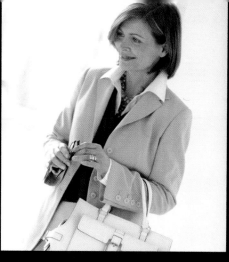
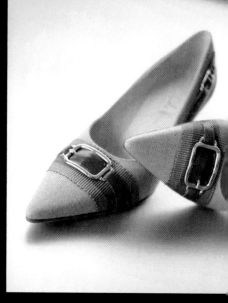
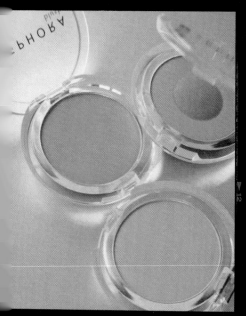
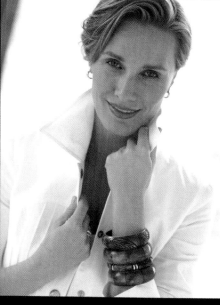
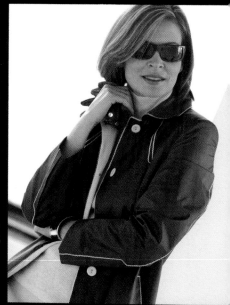
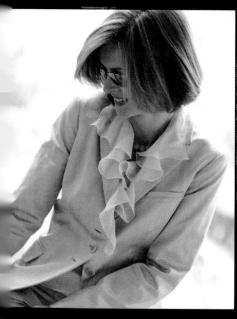
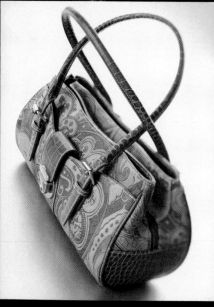
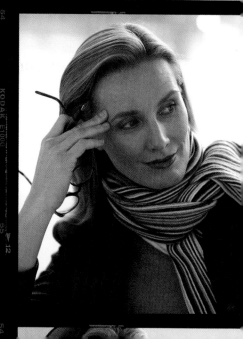
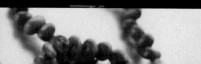

Contents

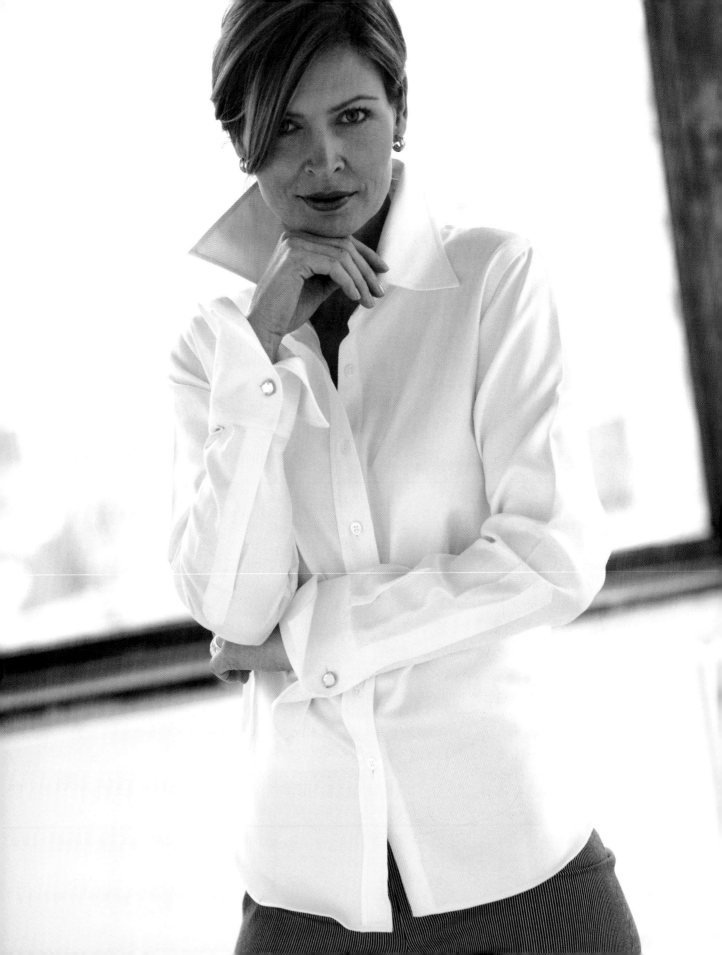

Introduction

Who is the grown-up girl? She is a forty-plus woman in the most unique position of any generation before her. She is living in unexplored territory where there is no precedent. Being in your forties, fifties, or sixties is no longer what it once was. Forty is now tagged "the new thirty." The forty-plus woman no longer fits the former labels of "mature," "middle-aged," or "older."

She is a grown-up girl.
She is empowered.
She wants to look her best.
She wants to feel her best.
She wants to project her best.
She wants to live her best.

She is a complex, distinctive individual, who is far from being on the downside of life. Turning forty, fifty, or sixty is not about getting older, it's about getting better. I know. I am one of the vast numbers of women who are dealing with the various aspects of aging on a daily basis. But instead of looking at aging as a negative, I look at it as an opportunity. We have lived long enough to know who we are. We have experienced enough to know what we like. We are opinionated, smart, and sassy. We are hardly the same at forty-plus that our mothers and grandmothers were. We want to approach aging with style and grace. We want to invest in our well-being. We don't need to look twenty.

The forty-plus woman no longer looks, acts, or realizes she is older. She has the choice to be young at heart, in body, and in mind. Unlike the generations before her, she has the ability to control many of her aging issues.

But she needs guidance, and to date there is none. Pundits say if it makes you feel good that's all that matters. How wrong they are!

Many women over forty are walking around revealing skin that begs to be covered, wearing clothing suited for their daughters, combing hair that cries for updating, and applying lipstick beyond their lipline for that trendy "pouty" mouth. They blame hormonal changes for their extra weight and PMS for cynical attitudes.

In many cases, while trying to appear younger, they are actually making themselves look and act older, and often foolish. Despite all the books, articles, and television segments on the subject, no one is pointing to the obvious. No one is telling the truth.

The media is aiming their messages at the eighteen to thirty-nine year olds. *The Grown-Up Girl's Guide to Style* is the book every forty-plus woman needs because it is the first book that gives honest solutions to problems that pertain specifically to a new generation wanting answers.

The New Forty-Plus Generation

Forty-plus is an age of opportunity.

Oprah turned fifty and continues to change the lives of women daily.

Sheryl Crow and Melissa Etheridge taught us you can still rock 'n roll through cancer.

Diane Keaton won the Golden Globe for Best Actress for her performance in *Something's Gotta Give*.

Goldie Hawn became a "glam-ma" for the first time.

Madonna opted for English proper over her leather-and-chains attire.

In *The Grown-Up Girl's Guide to Style* I will:

- Take you on an incredible self-improvement journey.

- Share my years of experience with you, as a professional and as a woman.

- Teach you everything the new over-forty woman needs to know.

- Give you insight into all phases of style and fashion.

- Show you how to balance the very important line between current and appropriate.

- Teach you about *selective revelation*, my most important fashion secret.

- Guide you through the incredible new world of beauty, both cosmetically and medically.

- Expose you to the advantages of a positive attitude.

- Bring some of the leading experts right into your home.

- Share lessons of life with you that will change the way you think about aging.

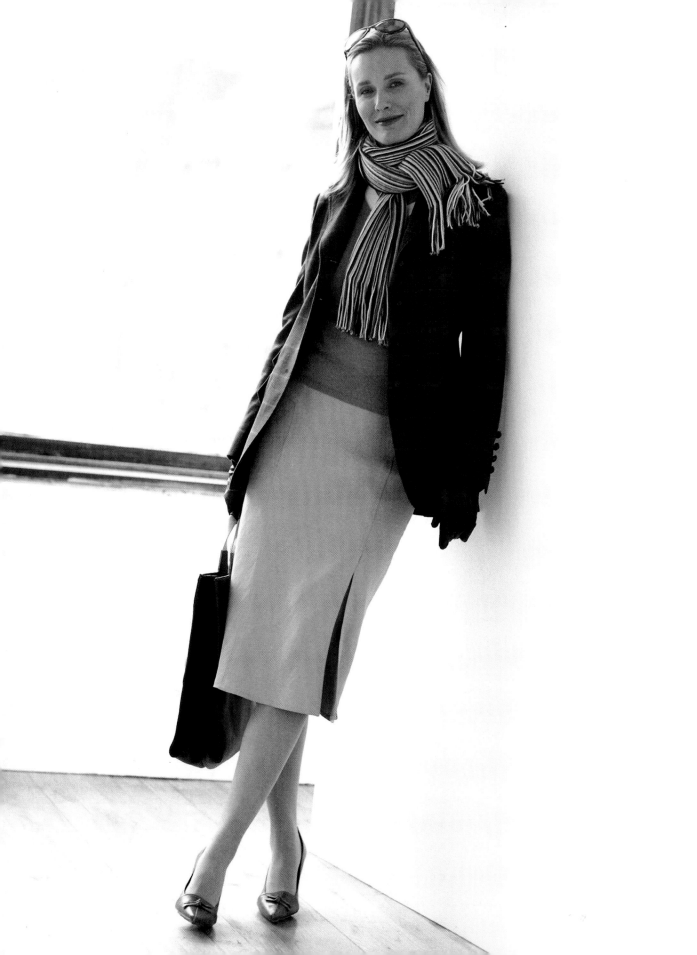

Together we will work on your mind, body, and appearance. I will give you honest answers to all your questions. I am not only concerned with helping you find just the right outfit for any event; I am concerned with every aspect of your physical and emotional well-being. Once we turn forty, it's not as simple as choosing what color lipstick to wear. It's putting together the entire package to make us stylish, fit, sexy, healthy, and happy.

I will challenge what fashion and beauty experts have been preaching for years. I might make some women angry, and others defensive, but those who listen will change the way they feel and look.

The Journey

This time of life can be your best if you make the necessary adjustments. The problem is most women are not addressing the changes that need to be made. They read fashion, health, and lifestyle books and magazines, but only a fraction of the advice pertains to them. Television shows are afraid to take a stand, so they waffle when they should be openly critical. Afraid to turn off advertisers, they say almost everything is okay if it makes you feel good. WRONG, WRONG, WRONG. Yes, you can do whatever you want, but my question to you is why would you want to do anything that makes you look foolish, inappropriate, or older? Why would you want to look like you are trying too hard? Designers don't design to make you look good, they design to sell merchandise. If we look foolish, how can we feel good?

How can we always look, feel, and be our best? The answer lies in finding the happy medium between the young trendy foolish looks and the boring frumpy "I give up" looks. It lies between the pamphlets' write-up on cosmetic procedures and the reality of having them. We should develop realistic and healthy eating habits rather than rely on diet books. We must get motivated to move our bodies in any way we can. It is essential to surround ourselves with positive influences, always moving forward. We need knowledge, and I am going to provide you with that education. I am going to give you what you want, need, and deserve.

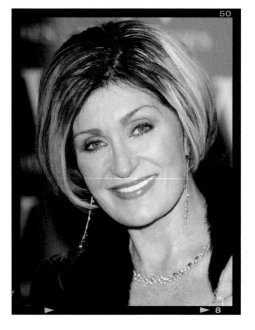

Sharon Osbourne does grown-up girl rock 'n' roll better than anyone.

I have adjusted my style and beauty routine over the years as my body changed. I am still fashionable and still think like I am thirty, even though I can no longer dress like I am. I watch women everywhere and am constantly amazed at their attempts to dress like they are twenty, only to look silly, and sometimes even worse than if they did nothing at all. I see them going to extremes with cosmetic dermatology treatments and plastic surgery, applying over-the-top makeup, wearing hairstyles that are either too young or too matronly, and dressing to reveal what needs to be covered. Some give up and give in to lifestyle choices that are no longer healthy. Others settle for less when they should be pursuing more. Far too many think they are too old, when they are actually just right.

I have come to the conclusion that grown-up living is a compromise between what's appropriate and what's right for you. At forty, Lisa Kudrow is that same free-spirited love child we came to know on *Friends*. Look at Sharon Osbourne; she is an advocate of cosmetic treatments and plastic surgery, wears cool trends, and adds bold streaks to her hair and she looks incredible. She has balanced the rock-and-roll look that fits her lifestyle with what works for her body. Diane Keaton, who is a naturalist, loves kooky clothing, and always creates her own style. She covers her liabilities with gloves and high necklines and yet allows her creativity to shine with cutting-edge eyewear and vintage accessories. Christie Brinkley at fifty still looks like the goddess next door with her fresh, wholesome style in both fashion and makeup. She has adjusted her look without losing it. Katherine Hepburn never lost her gender-bender style or her strong-willed outlook. Her classic turtlenecks and trouser pants worked for her well into her nineties. Her progressive thinking changed the way many females felt about themselves as women. Eleanor Roosevelt and Golda Meier used their ambition and intelligence to make a difference in public life. They taught prior generations of women that brains are as important as looks.

We are fortunate to live in an era of limitless options—to look, feel, and be fabulous way beyond forty. We don't need to think like our grandmothers. There is not a chronological age that now determines we are past our prime. Our prime is a state of mind.

I am recommending that you open yourself to the possibilities of changes in your style, beauty, health, and attitude. Below are some of the myths that kept previous generations from being ageless.

- You've earned the right to do whatever you want.
- You can't wear long hair past forty.

Kate has one of the freshest looks in Hollywood and yet sometimes even she gets it wrong: too much color, too many trends, simply too young a look. Did she raid her daughter's closet?

- Fashion and beauty are not as important as you get older.

- The younger the outfit, the younger you will look.

- If you've got it, flaunt it.

- You can never be too rich or too thin.

Wrong, wrong, wrong!

We are bombarded with ideas on how to look and feel younger. We can no longer depend on our friends for guidance, for they, too, are searching. The mistakes we make are costly, both to our pocketbooks and our self-esteem. Otherwise why would women our age wear ultralow pants with cropped tops? Skin-tight stretch pants over big bums? Baggy turquoise polyester sweatsuits? Poodle hair or '60s eyeliner? Talk endlessly about body functions and health issues? Or hook themselves up to gimmicky machines to spot reduce? Why don't the experts, friends, and family come to their rescue? I can sum it up in three words . . . "Donald Trump's comb over." He is surrounded by the best of the best, so why isn't someone telling him?

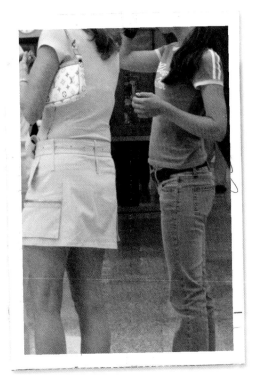

Even if you have great legs, why try to dress younger than your daughter?

Throughout my career in television and writing I have helped hundreds of thousands of women with their beauty and fashion needs. I have worked with celebrities, politicians, socialites, and homemakers. Regardless of their size or age, I have guided them to look and feel better. Now I am taking that thirty years of experience and directing it to a group in desperate need of direction. They want to find the balance between the extremes of the trends and the boredom of the staid and frumpy; the secrets to being forever ageless in both mind and manner; the lifestyle to keep forever healthy in attitude and body.

Past generations were compartmentalized into grandmothers, mothers, and career women; very few overlapped. A grandmother looked older than a career woman. A mother looked like a mother. There were rules about what you could or couldn't wear. Today the boundaries have blurred. The generations have blurred. Unfortunately, so have ideas of what's appropriate and what isn't.

The Grown-Up Girl's Guide to Style gives you the information you need to make your own choices based on your individual needs, not the needs advertisers tell you to have. We can look up to date without being trendy. We can be sexy without being foolish. We can be young without being youngsters. We are the new generation of women who appreciate who we are today, at this time in our life.

The Grown-Up Girl's Guide to Style will pull no punches. It will tell you what you need to hear, show you what you need to do, and explain how to achieve your goals. All I ask is that you leave your preconceptions at the door when reading this book. It's time to think anew.

Let's begin this incredible journey together.

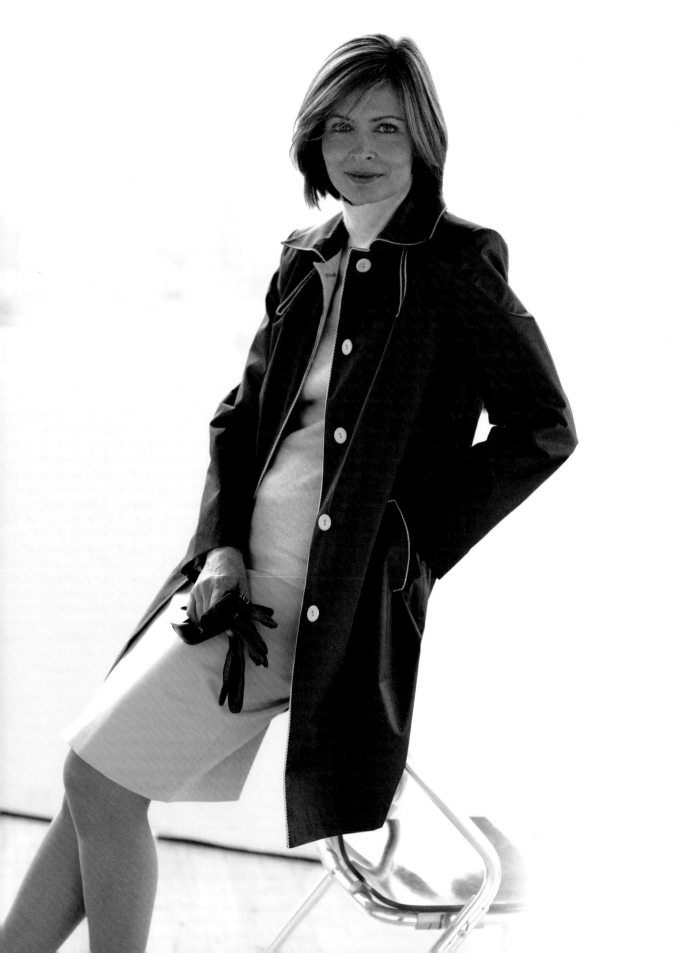

PART ONE

Fashion

The love affair between females and fashion begins the minute our infant feet hit the ground running in a new pair of Mary Jane shoes. Even at two years old we know a compliment when we hear one. We like the attention. We quickly make the association. We never outgrow the desire for flattery. Compliments are as ageless as we want to be. As we grow up it's imperative that our fashion styles grow with us. It doesn't have to grow older, just smarter. The compliments will follow.

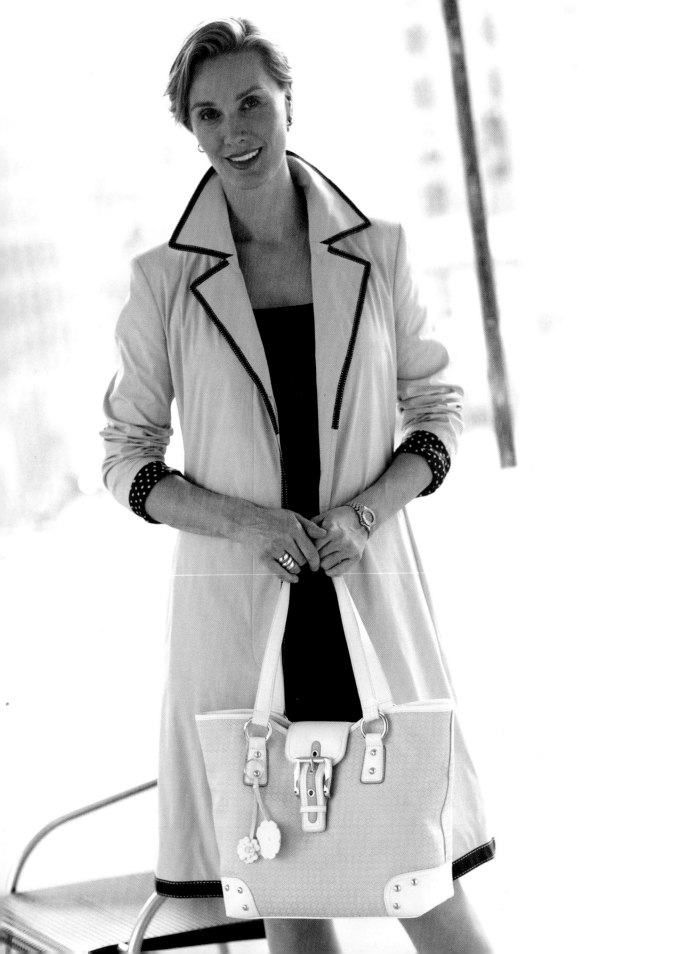

CHAPTER ONE

Style

What Is Style for the Grown-Up Girl?

Style is the most powerful word in fashion. It indicates that you've got it right. You are of the "elite" group that is in the know. You are savvy, smart, and have flair. You are confident.

My definition of style for the forty-plus woman is simply good taste, and everyone can have good taste. Some are born with style, but most of us learn it along the way. Good taste comes from knowledge. It comes from making mistakes, from being adventurous and yet balanced at the same time, and from wanting to look your best. It comes from a willingness to try. When you want to look good you can learn to look good. There is no magic as we are led to believe; there is only the right information. Did you learn to drive a car? Cook? Speak a foreign language? Then you can learn style. Why waste your time and money on the wrong things when you could be buying the right ones?

Good taste becomes even more important as we grow up. We have more decisions to make on what works and what doesn't. It becomes mandatory that we make the right ones. How do we do it? With knowledge: information empowers us and guides us. How we interpret that information becomes our own personal style.

Style is a little different for all of us. It's as unique as we are. It's the ultimate expression of who we are as women. But like everything else, style changes.

> *Our teen style was whatever our best friends wore.*
> *Our twenties style was what we could afford.*
> *In our thirties we experimented.*

In the forties came the style question . . .
"Does this look okay on me?"
In the fifties it's,
"Does this look too young or too old?"
And the sixties ask,
"Is this really appropriate?"
One of the greatest style icons of all time, Audrey Hepburn, said, "The more there
*   is, the less I want."*
That is grown-up girl's style.
Simplicity.

It's combining classic, contemporary, and personal elements. It's not about a head-to-toe Ralph Lauren outfit, or what's hot in the fall fashion issue of *Vogue.* It's not the latest runway look. It's about us. It's about the mix of a crisp, tailored, white cotton Gap shirt with a Michael Kors slim chocolate brown pencil skirt and brown suede pumps, or the way you wear an heirloom brooch on the neckline of a shirt. Grown-up girl style is the burnt red lipstick you have worn for years or the full, straight bangs that have been your signature. It's a way of dressing to express your good taste, your confidence, and your personality. Style is all about you.

By the time we reach forty we pretty much know who we are. We know what we like and what we don't. Our style is somewhat set, but then fashion changes come along and tempt us. This is where the quandary begins. In your twenties and thirties your only concerns were lifestyle and dress size. If you had the bucks and the body, you went for it. In the forties the criteria begin to change and continue to change dramatically. Having the budget and the body is no longer enough, we must also have the education. This education will open up a whole new fashion world to you. One that is exciting yet suitable. This knowledge will set you free from the pressure of trying to be "in" when the real importance is in being marvelously ageless.

Style Icons

We can learn a lot about style by looking at role models. Here are some of my favorites and the lessons I have learned from them.

GRACE KELLY
Always looked like a lady. Her classic beauty and style are as timeless today as they were years ago. She never went for trends, she went for exquisiteness.

SOPHIA LOREN

Still strikingly sexy without looking silly. She never gave up her big hair and yet it always looks right on her. She added a little weight and made it look voluptuous. Only those overdecorated eyeglasses detract from her beauty.

SELA WARD

A contemporary, relaxed Jacqueline Kennedy. Her look is simple and classic. Can you even imagine her dressed head-to-toe in animal print?

KIM BASINGER

Hollywood glamour that always makes you go right to the store and buy all new skin treatments. She has that flawless face we all dream of.

AMY BRENNEMAN

Makes me want to curl my hair and roll up the cuffs of my jeans. She is the perfect naturalist.

BARBRA STREISAND

Taught me that all faces do not need to look alike. Her nose sets her apart. She doesn't try to look like anyone else. She looks like Barbra and we like the way she looks.

LAUREN HUTTON

Proves that refreshing is youthful. Her clean, fresh face only looks better as she ages.

JACLYN SMITH

Made me want to copy her tailored style when she was a "Charlie's Angel" and I still do, all these years later.

KATE CAPSHAW

Teaches me the importance of youthful hair. Her style and color adjusts each year to keep her looking like she never ages.

JAYNE KENNEDY

Has stature. Her perfect posture allows her to carry a fuller figure with pure elegance.

MEREDITH VIERA

Proves that not everyone has to have plastic surgery to look good.

TINA TURNER AND SHARON OSBORNE

Show me that a little rock 'n' roll style still works if you do it with flair.

DIANE SAWYER

Proves that a great shirt, a pencil skirt, and high heels make one of our best outfits.

QUEEN NOOR OF JORDAN

Proves that elegance is always appropriate.

ANNETTE BENING

Really does seem to have it all in balance: a sexy husband, four children, and a career.

ELLEN DEGENERES

Shows me that you can be who you are, dress the way you want, and make it all work for you.

CATHERINE DENEUVE

Teaches me that when it comes to style, we can learn from the French. They buy quality, buy less, and keep it forever. Makes our trends look as silly as they sometimes are.

DEMI MOORE

Goes against my theory about showing too much skin. When your body looks like hers you get to do whatever you want.

JACQUELINE KENNEDY

Got it right all the time. I learned to ask myself why does something work? One look at how she dressed and you know. Simplicity.

CHER

Proves that the technology exists to make us look forever thirty, but why would we want to?

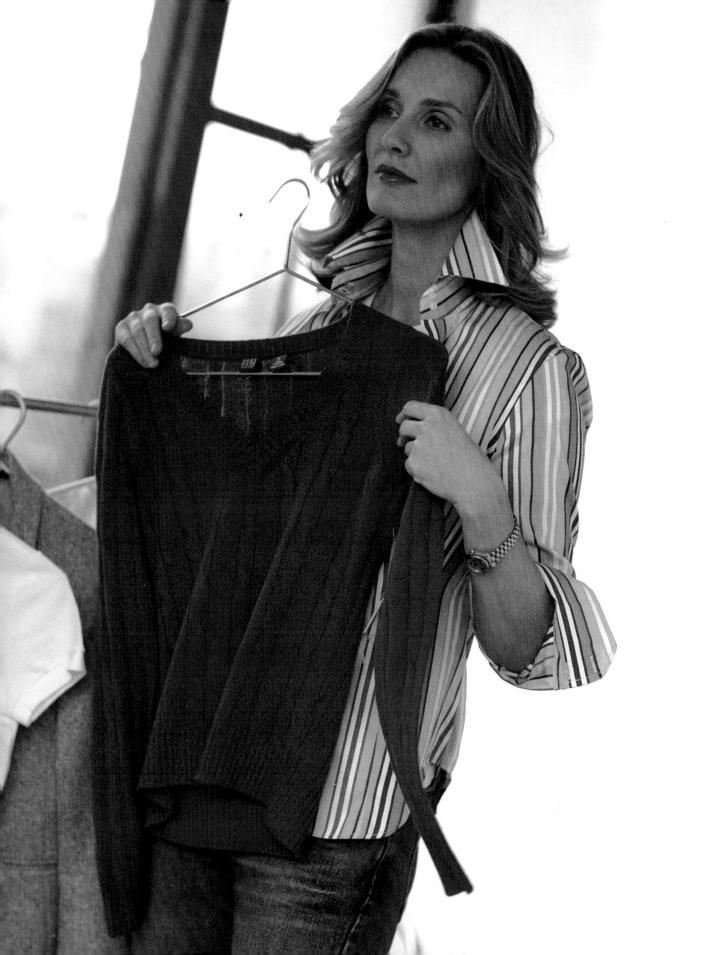

The Style Killer

I can put it in one word: *matron*. The dictionary defines matron as "a woman, especially a married woman of middle age or later, who has had children and is thought of as being mature, sensible, and of good social standing." Take it out of our vocabulary. Remove it from the dictionary. Erase it from your mind. The dictionary also defines it as "a woman who is a warden in a women's correctional institution." Leave the word there. We never, ever want to be associated with the word *matron*. Today's forty-plus woman is far from being a matron. And yet we all know of a few.

Most of my friends have evolved, but a few have gone in the wrong direction. They think old, talk old, act old, and dress old. They have given up. They would rather talk about what pills they are taking than what shoes they are buying. They live with what might have been, instead of what might be. They have fast-forwarded into old age, even though chronologically they are not there. They think of themselves as mature, way too mature for their own good.

I ask myself why? Is it easier to give up? Perhaps for them it is and yet when I look at them I realize that with just a few simple changes they could revert back to the youthful women they once were. Instead of taking advantage of all that is available to us in today's society, they live in the world of their mothers and grandmothers. Appropriate, to them, is acting their age, according to dictionary definitions from 1950. What has stunted their growth? If you think matron, you will be matronly. If you think young, you will be young. It starts first in your mind and works its way into your style.

The Style Checklist

What do you need to be stylish? You might think I would say a new jacket or a designer bag. Wrong. Style starts and ends in your head. The fashionable part of style comes from the inside out. Once we get the right mindset, the rest is a piece of cake.

Here is my checklist:

- The right attitude
- An open mind
- Courage to try new things
- The ability to break old habits
- The ability to look at your positives and negatives

- The insight to borrow from your style icons

- The courage to put your own individual twist on style

- The mindset to stay positive

- The desire to be interested in others

- The determination to never, ever get cynical

- The ability to keep up with fashion and adapt a little of it in your look

- The passion to always evolve

- The pride to care about the way you present yourself

- The ability to like yourself enough to make a difference

Now we can add the designer bag or the new jacket. Work on your mind first and your appearance second. The first will set you in motion for the other. It's time to get in motion.

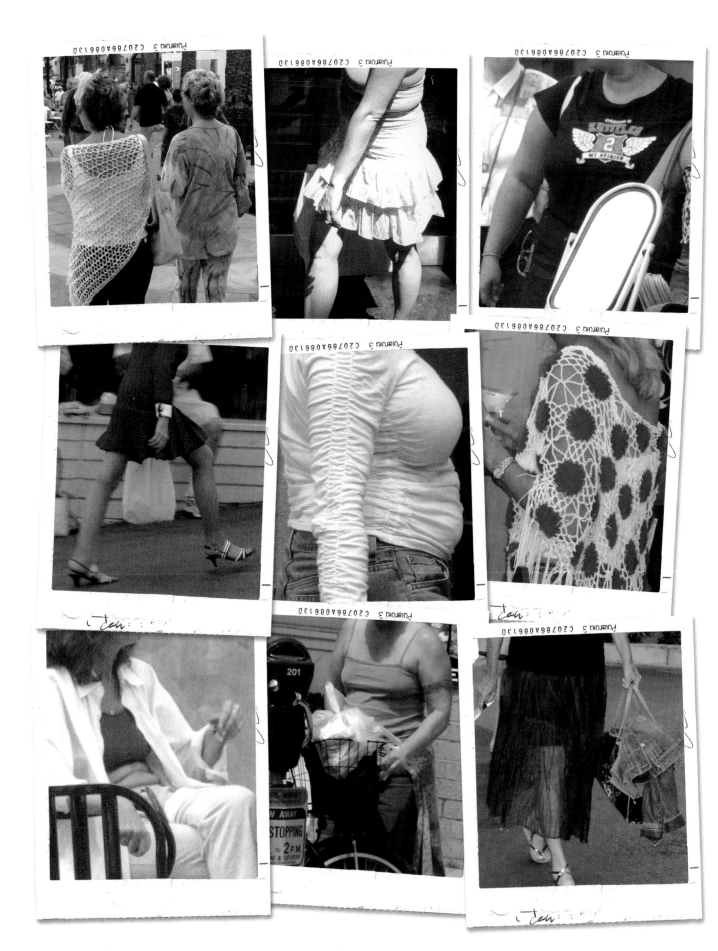

CHAPTER TWO

Fashion Disasters

For us it's not as often about what you do right as it is about what you do wrong. By the time we reach forty-plus we think we know what works. We know our figure assets and flaws. We have opinions on what colors are flattering. Many times we are right on target but often we are not. Then the target changes and sometimes we don't.

Loved those clingy tank tops in your thirties? You probably can't cling to them much longer. Do you have a closet full of studded jeans that always make you feel sexy? It's probably time to feel sexy without your studs. Your cutoff line may be at forty, it may be at fifty, but believe me, if it hasn't already arrived, it's on its way. You might be too busy to notice—but others will.

The stares that you take for compliments could be stares of disbelief. How do you know the difference? Sometimes the realization comes when you are in the dressing room trying on clothes and you feel a little foolish with your choices. It often hits when you see a teenager in the same pants as yours. Perhaps you find yourself shopping in the "mature" section of the department store because it's the only place where anything fits. Often you have to be hit over the head with a rude comment. The important thing is that you get hit. Here are some of the biggest mistakes that grown-up girls make. Don't pooh-pooh them—read them and then take a serious look in your closet and drawers and most importantly, in the mirror.

Disaster #1—Nakedness: How Dare You Bare

The number one fashion mistake our age group makes is baring too much skin. Many of the clothes offered in stores encourage this bareness. Why is showing skin risky?

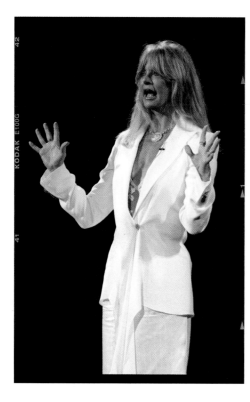

Her smile lights up a room. Her neckline makes it buzz, but not for the right reasons.

You may be thin, and toned, and that may be enough—or it might not. You must also look at your skin texture. Skin texture changes, especially white skin. Skin with color is the exception; Asian and black skin usually has a good five- to ten-year advantage. Plus-size women also have better skin texture, but when they reveal skin they also reveal weight. I say retain the mystery. Body tone changes. I don't care how well you take care of yourself, most of us, even Goldie, need a little more covering.

GROWN-UP GIRL'S COVER-UP RULE:

Show only what you want others to see. When in doubt, if you can grab and jiggle it, cover it.

FASHION MYTH: "YOU'VE EARNED THE RIGHT TO DRESS HOWEVER YOU WANT."

Yes, indeed you have, but why would you want to if it doesn't make you look your best?

What is it with all the body revelation? I understand it if you're twenty, or even thirty, but when I see the forty- and fifty-year-olds dressing bare, bare, bare, I say why? Do they really think this makes them look young? Don't they realize that they look like they are trying to imitate Britney Spears? Britney went from fresh and wholesome to sex symbol. It works for her. It doesn't work for us. I am not saying cover everything. If you have areas that are not affected by aging, reveal them! Otherwise cover or draw attention away from age-bearing sites. It's called *selective revelation*.

Nakedness is beautiful on a lovely young body. It is foolish on anyone else. It doesn't matter how much plastic surgery you've had or how toned you are, there is a cutoff point for baring your tummy, a deadline for baring your breasts, a time limit for going sleeveless. Just because you feel comfortable showing too much skin doesn't mean you should.

Are we past perfection? Absolutely not! Perfection comes in knowing when to stop revealing. Perfection is playing up your assets and hiding your liabilities. We have heard it over and over with dressing-thin tips. Now it's time to hear it over and over for dressing right. Barbara Walters wore an asymmetrical off-the-shoulder dress to the Emmys. She revealed a little of one shoulder and the top of one arm. Her long gloves covered all the rest. She looked sexy at over seventy. She didn't look naked.

How long has it been since you have made a personal body inspection? Really, who even wants to? For our educational purposes, we have to start with a diagnosis. In order to know how to dress we must first understand what our assets and liabilities are. They are not the same as they were ten or fifteen years ago, but then we're not the same. We've improved and we will be even better once we take stock of what's "hot" and what's not.

That former suntan has reappeared as freckles that are no longer cute. Did anyone tell us that "lizard texture" would show up in anything other than an expensive purse? Those fast-food stops for the kids that once accumulated trash inside our cars have now accumulated trash inside our thighs and buttocks in the form of cellulite. Pregnancies and weight gains left extra skin behind as a not-so-gentle reminder. But no one will know if we cover. I don't mean head-to-toe covering. I mean being selective about what you put on view.

Regardless of how much you diet or exercise, unless you are into surgery, suction, and injections, certain areas need immediate attention. You can modify them somewhat with products and treatments, or you can simply apply makeup or dress in a way that detracts. Diet and exercise make you look and feel better but still don't give you permission to reveal what begs to be covered.

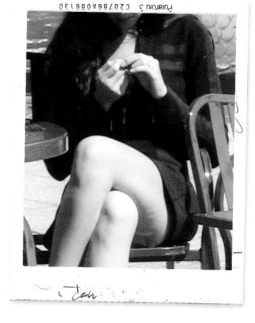

Selective Revelation

Look closely and be honest—you don't have to share this information with anyone. Then, adopt selective revelation. My definition of selective revelation is finding your best body areas and revealing enough of them to give the impression that what you cover is in the same condition. It's a great little secret, a little fooling device that doesn't hurt anyone. Here are some suggestions:

Obviously, she doesn't realize how much she's giving away.

- **Nice shoulders:** Choose one-shoulder dresses or tops that reveal just a little shoulder, but a little is all you need to make the impression.

- **A chest that hasn't seen the sun:** Wear your blouses slightly more opened; your V-necks a little deeper, your scoop necks a little wider. You don't need to cover spots and dots like the majority of us sun worshipers.

- **Attractive hands:** Add a beautiful, bold ring.

- **A slim torso:** Wear body-conscious clothing, *not tight*, just skimming your curves.

- **A great tush:** Tailor your pants to fit perfectly.
- **Toned calves:** Wear high heels. Keep your skirt lengths appropriate but tailor in a slit at your best zone.
- **A pretty face:** Show off your bone structure with turtlenecks, notable collars, exquisite earrings, and the perfect hairstyle.
- **A small waist:** Belt it in with an important belt.

Think of the spotlights used in theater. They focus on what they want to highlight. A single book on a table will have its own key light. Use your selective revelations to highlight where you want your focus. We don't need head-to-toe fabric. We want to create mystery. We don't want to look like we are hiding anything. Selective revelation is achieving the balance between covering and revealing.

Body areas that exhibit age the least are usually the back, shoulders, forearms, and legs below the knee. Use these to your advantage. Coverage is not a negative. A slim, high-neck, long-sleeve dress that hits midknee can be sexier than a sheer, low-cut slip dress that reveals all.

THE SLEEVELESS SITUATION

Don't wear sleeveless.

Don't wear short sleeves.

Just don't. Unless you have perfect arms.

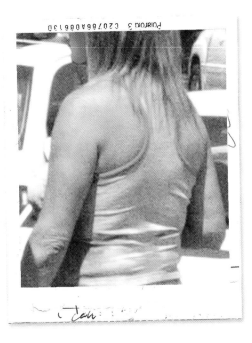

If you are screaming, "But I live in a hot climate," stop kvetching. So you work out and your arms have real, honest-to-goodness definition when you flex? This does not mean they can handle sleeveless tops. Do you flex your arms while you are driving a car, having a conversation, or grocery shopping? I don't think so. I know of very few women over forty who have good upper arms, and even fewer who have elbows worth revealing. One of my friends argues with me on a regu-

The racer-back style was first designed for real athletes. The weekend athlete quickly adopted the look. How did we ever let it venture out on the streets?

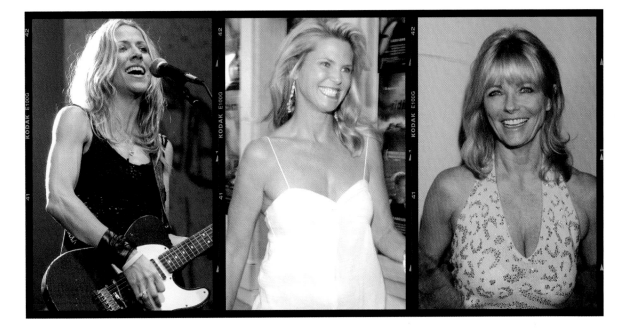

Okay, okay, I know of Sheryl Crow and Madonna. Their arms are definitely sleeveless worthy.

She's got the face. She's got the body. She just doesn't have the upper arms.

If that animal wrap was placed up on her shoulders we would never know that Cheryl's arms have passed the sleeveless era. The importance of a good wrap is that it covers.

lar basis about this theory. She flexes her arms for me—in her sleeveless tops—and they do look good. Then she relaxes and talks with her hands. Her arms are no longer flexed, and they are no longer sleeveless worthy. She only looks at them when she flexes. Everyone else looks at them all the time. What's so great about sleeveless if it doesn't flatter you?

For shirt or T-shirt coverage try the coolness of cotton or linen. They breathe and are every bit as cool as sleeveless. Synthetics can stifle. Long sleeves pushed up or rolled below the elbow allow you to be comfortable yet chic.

Can't find anything long-sleeved in the spring or summer? Shop for tissue-weight cotton long sleeves in the cooler months. Keep looking, they are there. Cruisewear comes to the stores in early January, and so should you. You will find some of your best summer items in the dead of winter. By planning ahead you can assemble a fabulous collection of cool, long-sleeved dresses, shirts, and T-shirts to push or roll up all summer long.

Don't wear shorts! Replace them immediately with cropped pants. They reveal a little ankle, which is usually a good thing. Any cellulite, broken veins, or lumpy texture should never see the light of day. Not even the longer shorts make my cut unless you have beyond fabulous legs. Have you ever really looked at a knee? Knees were not beautiful when we were twenty. At forty and over . . . you get the picture.

Katie Couric has great legs, including her knees. She wears fabulous high heel shoes and crosses them perfectly as she does her interviews. Mary Hart has insured her legs for millions. Did your legs pass your body inspection?

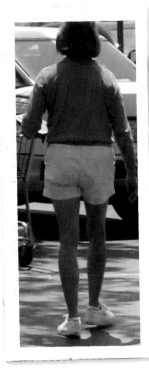

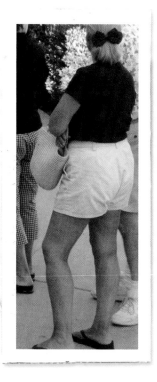

Believe me, it's never hot enough to go public with shorts. Shorts are for those involved in sports where they are required. You can't exercise in shorts without revealing underwear, not to mention your body parts. Those lycra shorts that cling might look good on a bicyclist from the back but have you looked at them from the front? Have you noticed where they cling?

Not even the bow can take our eyes off of legs that should be covered. Keep white colors by your face where they flatter instead of fatter.

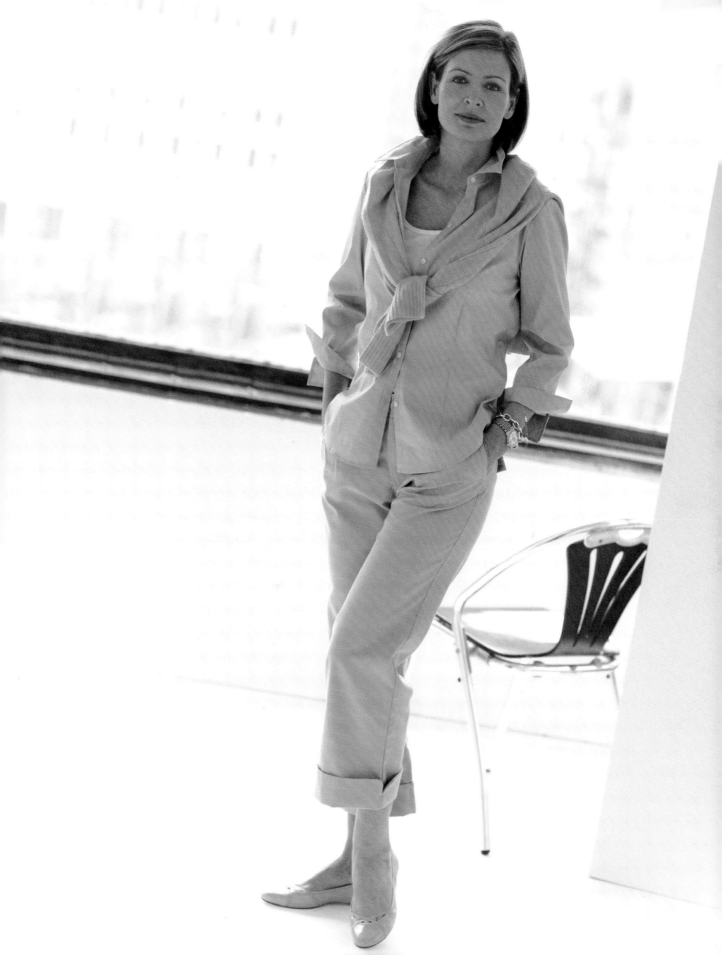

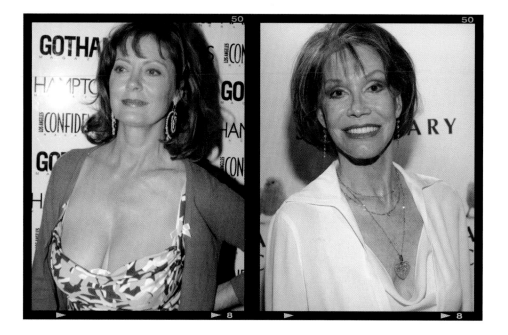

What happened to support? Susan could use a little . . . or perhaps a lot. She has wonderful skin and fabulous breasts—it's just that they have changed location and nobody is telling her.

Mary always makes us laugh. We like her looking sweet, not inappropriately sexy. Her smile is enough for us.

BAN THE BOOBS

Save your breasts for your significant other. The public doesn't need to see them. *Cleavage* is a word that must be banished from most of our vocabularies. We don't need a bra that pushes our breasts together, we need one that supports them. Keep your blouses buttoned above your bra, keep your V-necks higher, give away your wide scoop necks or off-the-shoulder tops or wear them with a high cut tank underneath and burn your strapless. Use J.Crew's long-sleeved tissue-weight T-shirts under revealing tops. They stylishly conceal without adding bulk.

Sure Kim Cattrall and Heather Locklear get away with baring their breasts. They have incredible breasts. They also have a "breast-revealing" celebrity lifestyle. The paparazzi at red carpet events love breasts of all kinds. A little revelation guarantees you good photo placement. But we are not fighting for paparazzi attention. The only attention we want is the right kind and too much revelation will guarantee you just the opposite. Just because you've got them, doesn't mean you need to flaunt them.

When Matt Lauer asked Tina Turner on the *Today* show if he was going to see her famous legs on her upcoming tour, she replied "A little. At 65 there are different ways to do it." Tina Turner knows the importance of the placement of skirt length. She gets it.

Any skirt that inches above the knees must go. They become minis when you sit. If you wore minis in the sixties, you can't wear them now, including wrap skirts, or as I call them "gap skirts." Have you ever been able to sit in one without tugging? And getting out of a car? Don't even try!

Our new genteel skirt length is skimming the knee or longer. There are really only two skirts that always flatter: the pencil (or slim) skirt and the A-line.

Regardless of your size, if you buy a pencil or slim skirt that falls straight over your tush you can look good in a size 6 or a 16. It's all about the fit. Anything that curves in below your bottom is too tight. Don't worry about the labeled size, worry about how it looks on you. If you have good legs use a small slit to show them off. You can have your tailor close up a thigh-high slit on a revealing skirt or add a small slit to a conservative one.

The A-line skirt is the most forgiving skirt of all because it eases over your hips and thighs. Buy one that skims easily, which means buy a bigger size and have the waist taken in if necessary.

Choose a skirt fabric that doesn't cling. If you want to wrap yourself in Saran Wrap, be my guest, but do it for your significant other in the privacy of your home. For that other cling, static cling, use one of the antistatic sprays. They are a wardrobe stylist's staple. A little spray under your skirt not only gets your attention (no wonder Marilyn Monroe stood above that air shaft) but it prevents unflattering cling.

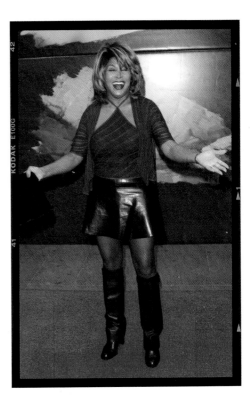

Between her boots and her skirt hemline, Tina Turner shows very little leg, but what she shows is good. Notice the placement of her two tops. They reveal some without revealing all: strategic and appropriate.

Bias-cut skirts *They cling, shift, and look good on the hanger, but not on the body. This is a styling gimmick that we can leave in the stores.*

Long skirts

- *A slim long skirt with a slit can work if the fabric is solid, subtle, and sophisticated.*
- *A menswear tweed or stripe works, an embossed floral does not. Be careful you don't look like you're wearing your sofa.*
- *A summer floral in a soft cotton, gauze, or linen is pretty as long as the color and print don't overpower you.*

Midcalf skirts *This is a sophisticated length with high-heeled pumps or boots. The secret is to always match the color of your skirt hem with your opaque nylons (if you are wearing nylons) and your shoes. This elongates your body.*

Full, dirndl, pleated, or circle skirts *These look like schoolgirl skirts. However long it's been since you graduated is how long you should have avoided these shapes.*

Ruffled skirts *One single ruffle in a summer skirt is okay, two or more is frumpy.*

Shoes *are crucial for the right skirt look. They must be contemporary. In the summer a heeled mule or strappy sandal always works. In the winter, choose a heeled boot. The key is heels. Only someone with a tall, slim torso can wear long skirts with flat heels without looking frumpy.*

FASHION MYTH: "SHORT WOMEN CAN'T WEAR LONG SKIRTS."

They can and should, as long as they match everything from head to toe: that includes top, pants or skirt, belt, any leg covering, and shoes in all the same color. Always add some type of heel for extra height. The all-one-color, or monochromatic look is both elegant and elongating.

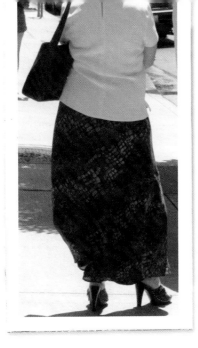

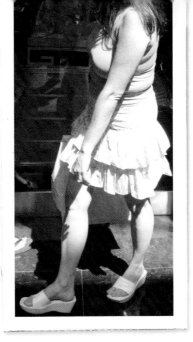

A few inches shorter and a contempo-rary shoe and bag would have said "twenty-first century" rather than "eighties."

What was she thinking? Ruffles do not balance out rolls. It's too short, too tight, and there's too much going on.

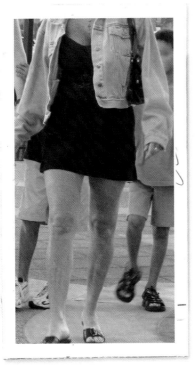

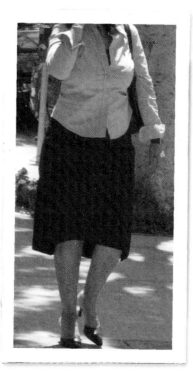

She's almost got the right idea— classic denim jacket, nice access-ories, black summer dress. She just doesn't have enough of it.

Uneven hems can strategically hide leg issues.

Evaluate your legs and adjust your stocking choices accordingly. The better the quality of the skin on your legs, the sheerer your nylons can be. Now we understand why they invented opaques: they cover and slim.

Sheer blouses and tops only work if you promise not to remove your sweater or jacket in public. Colorful and amusing print bras can make you wear a secretive smile on your face as long as only you know you're wearing them. Courtney Cox gets away with a lacy black bra under her white shirt. Beyoncé looks sexy showing her animal print cami through her sheer black sleeveless tank. We are not Courtney or Beyoncé, in age or lifestyle.

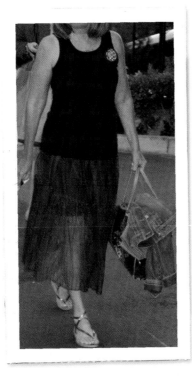

The right idea ended just above her knees! A cotton legging to the hem of the skirt would have made this worthy of going public.

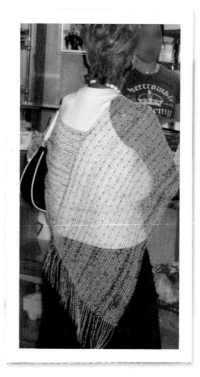

This lacy poncho is the perfect way to wear sheer. The delicate weave gives just enough coverage to make sleeveless a possibility.

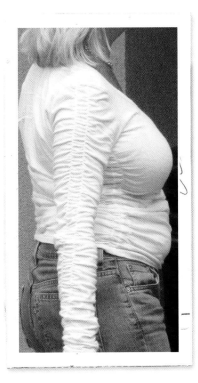

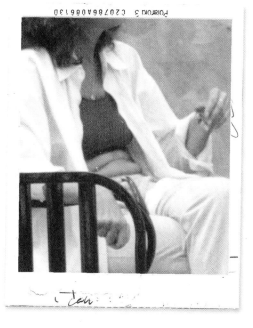

Body-hugging clothing is almost as bad as naked. You might not see the skin, but you sure get the idea. Full figures look best in fabulous shirts.

I'm sure when she stands up this outfit looks a lot better. However, she's sitting and revealing. Fastening the two middle buttons would keep her secrets secret.

BELLY ACHES

Crop-tops, low-riding pants, and drop-waist skirts reveal naked tummies. I think they should come with a warning label "Wear at Your Own Exposure." It doesn't count to hold your tummy in when you make the decision. If your forties are fading, don't even think it, let alone reveal it. Teri Hatcher might look sexy, we will only look silly. If a trend is really hot with the teenagers it is probably not right for us. If you must, wear your PJ bottoms lower and add a mini-top—in the privacy of your bedroom. It's perfect for sleeping—not perfect for the light of day.

I feel the hardest item of clothing to buy is a swimsuit. Trying on suits in that dressing room, we all have the same experience. This one makes us look too fat, that one makes us look too short, and another makes us look plain silly. With swimsuits everything hangs out.

Unless you are totally toned and smooth-skinned, the days of parading around in a swimsuit should be left behind. Really, we *only* need a swimsuit for real swimming or hot tub lounging (and I don't recommend hot tubs because nothing dries your skin out more). Short, romantic hot tub interludes—okay. Lounging—do it on a chaise.

So for swimsuits? Give them up unless you are in the pool or ocean, actually swimming, or you look like Kim Cattrall from the neck down. "Her body looks great for her age" is not what you want to hear. Save your body for under the covers with your favorite partner. It is not a requirement to be nearly naked for admission to the beach.

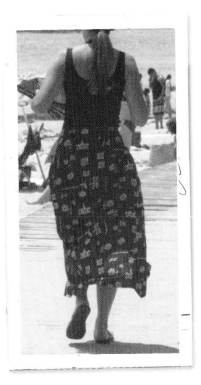

There are many very attractive beach or pool alternatives. Rolled up khakis with a big white shirt, and a fabulous straw hat cover up any suit with flair. Juicy Couture makes linen, drawstring pants that pair delightfully with long-sleeved T-shirts. Gauzy, cotton skirts with tank tops underneath an unbuttoned, sheer long-sleeved shirt with the sleeves rolled are airy, cool, and charming. A flowing cotton pareo knotted at the side paired with a wrap blouse are grown-up summer style.

When we must wear a suit it should be either a solid, basic one-piece without gimmicks or a two-piece tank top with a bottom that covers ours. Prints attract more attention. If you body is worthy of attention please indulge. If you are looking for the least obvious way to move from lounge chair to pool, do it in subtle solid color. Yes, that one large vertical stripe running down the side of your suit will make you look taller, but it will also emphasize your body shape. Red might be your most flattering color, but do you want it bringing all eyes on your torso?

A soft flowing cotton skirt lets you move around the beach or pool in private style.

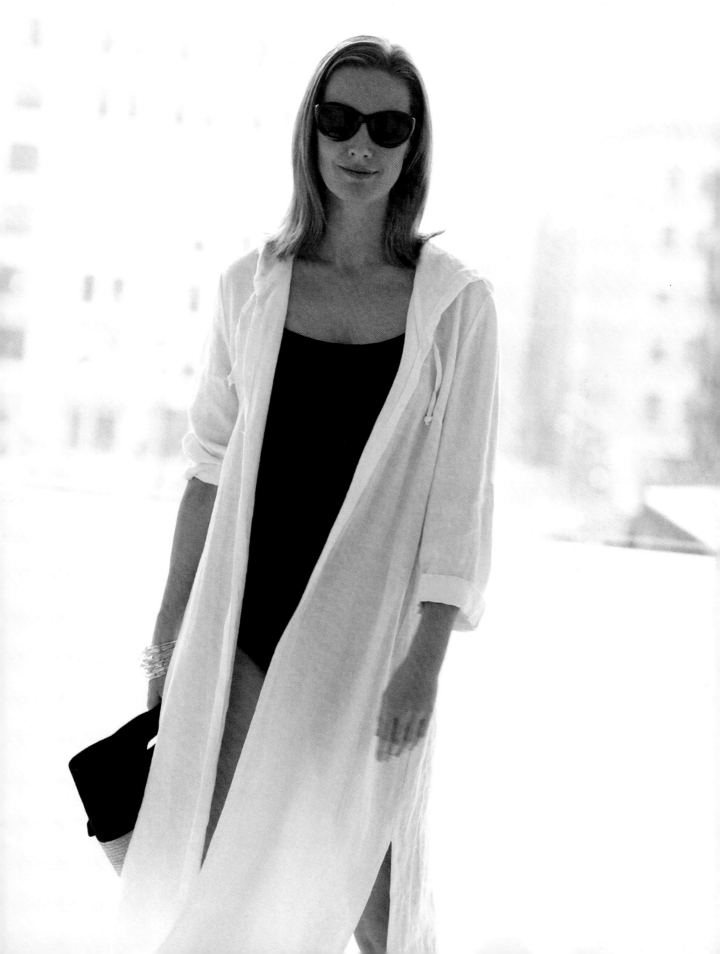

NIGHTTIME GIVEAWAYS

What happens when the sun goes down? Nighttime does not mean our boobs have to rise to the occasion. I know it's hard to find something for evening wear that doesn't reveal, but keep looking. Why do designers think nighttime is baretime?

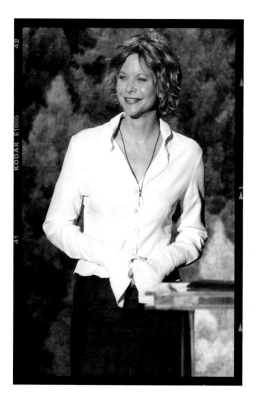

It always amazes me to go to a black-tie party event and see women I thought had great bodies revealing that they really don't. Strapless may be in style, but it's not the style we need if we don't have a smooth chest that has never seen the bright, damaging sun. A hollowness between our breasts may look sexy on Kate Hudson but not on us. Our upper arms might jiggle as we dance, but no one has to know it if we don't show them.

We have to change our way of thinking. Nighttime wear can be sexy without us being nearly naked. Nothing gives away age faster than uncovered, revealing evening attire. Don't look at the dress; look at how you look in the dress. Don't compete with the very young . . . out-style them.

Good evening choices

A long black slit skirt with a beaded top, cashmere sweater, starched white shirt, shrug or short, fitted jacket.

Classic evening suits, statement-making jackets, and pants or skirts, are perfect in beautiful wools, satins, or taffetas. They crave to be accessorized with glamorous touches.

Meg has the wholesome, adorable, girl-next-door evening look covered. Literally.

Opposite: Black sheer camouflages more than white sheer. Look closely before you purchase sheer. Veiling may or may not give you the cover you need.

The classic long-sleeved, slim, neutral color dress that falls gracefully to the floor. Pair this with a long, fitted evening coat and you command attention.

Tuxedos with skirts or pants are covered elegance.

Adding high heels, black sheer nylons, striking jewelry, a gemstone or pearl-decorated belt, gloves, a small charming bag, and captivating fragrance will elevate a black skirt and top to elegant evening status.

GROWN-UP GIRL'S EVENING WEAR RULE:

Create your evening wardrobe with separates. Buy unique pieces as you find them, not as you need them.

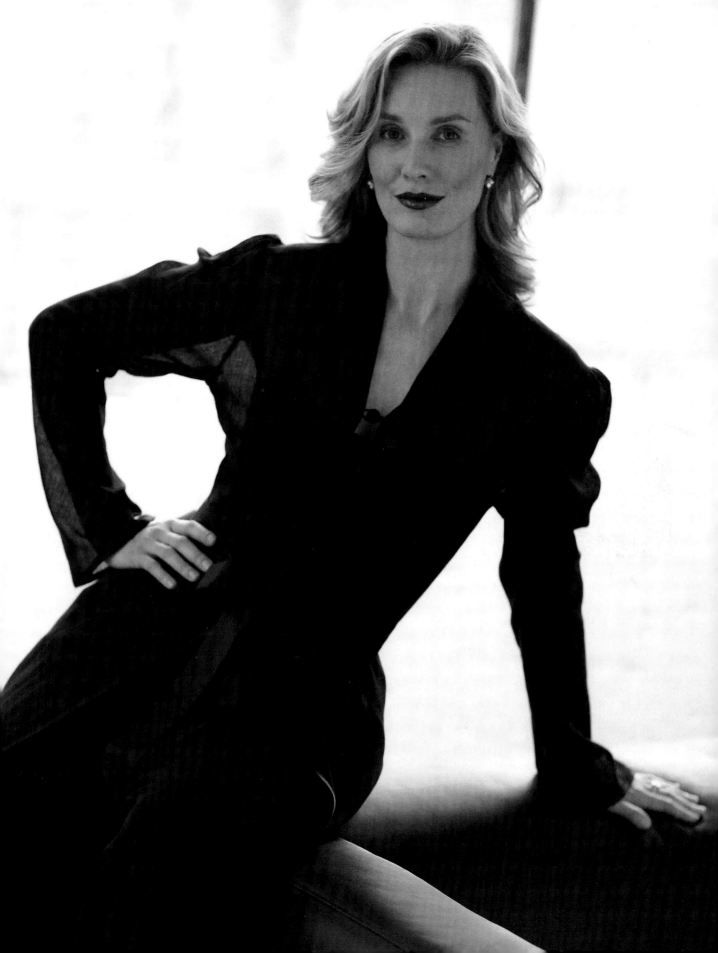

Now that I have told you many things that you can't do, you must be wondering what you can do. Plenty, and it all begins in the privacy of your bedroom. This is the one time where you can be as naked as you want. Sometimes, though, we go the opposite way. Why do grown-up women change into Aunt Ida when they get ready for bed?

What does your sleepwear look like? If it's an oversized T-shirt with a cute saying on the front, it's time to go shopping. If it's something you have worn for years, it's time to throw it out. Sloppy, dull, or frumpy must not be the words to describe what we sleep in.

If you like a sweet look, try a feminine nightgown with a matching robe. A pair of flannel PJs in menswear fabrics can be sweet and sexy if you put a lacy camisole or a ribbed tank under the top and leave it unbuttoned.

If you like sexy you can do all the things with sleepwear that you can't do in public. Bare, bare, bare if you and your mate prefer. Leather and wild animal prints? Not for the light of day, but in the candlelight of night? Whatever turns you on. All the nakedness rules go out the door when you close the one on your bedroom.

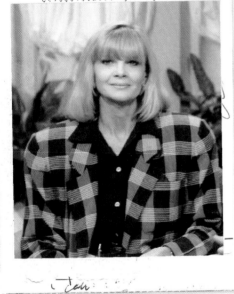

Honest, it only looks like I play for the NFL. In the late '80s I was cohost of the Fashion Channel. They actually paid me to wear this jacket.

Disaster #2—Trends

We watch television for fashion. The stars' unique styles give us material for conversation. They do not, however, dictate our style. Fashion has been my professional life for over thirty years. No one loves the trends more than I do. At one point in my career I wouldn't even think of wearing anything that wasn't cutting-edge. I have several embarrassing photos of myself to prove it!

Now as I try on the sheer summer slip dress I saw in *InStyle* magazine I realize that as much as I adore the look on Katie Holmes, I don't adore it on myself. I exercise, eat healthy, and count my calories. Yet as I change I find the need to change my style. It's not a compromise; it's just a very positive adjustment.

A trend is what the fashion world does to get us back in the stores spending. That's why they change every season. How else could we keep the designers employed? The time has come to return to the classics: a good suit, a great dress, a crisp, lightly starched shirt, a flattering skirt, a pair of blue jeans without adornments, and a closet full of wonderful cashmere sweaters. The Audrey Hepburn, Jacqueline Kennedy, Gwyneth Paltrow basics—these items are timeless, ageless, graceful, and flattering.

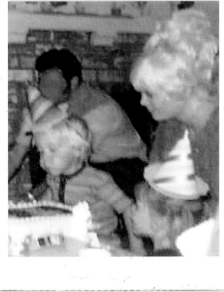

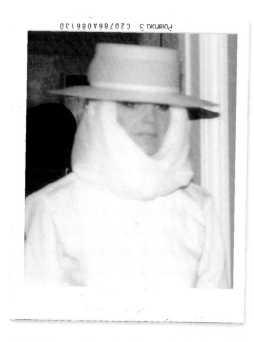

My three-year-old son celebrated his birthday with friends, a cake, and colorful paper hats. I celebrated it with a high-fashion hairpiece. In retrospect, I probably should have worn a paper hat.

No, I did not work as a beekeeper. I actually put this outfit together to wear to a cutting-edge summer fashion show. This was my "bored with mainstream" era.

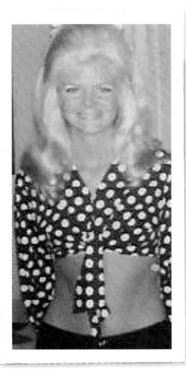

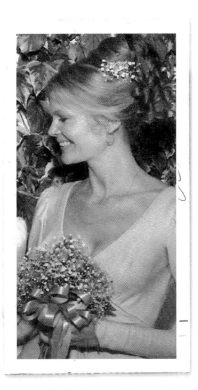

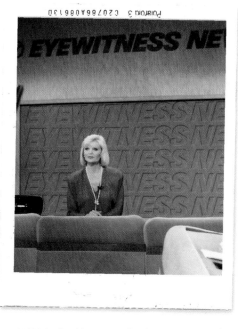

My style as I approached twenty was what I considered "hot" at the time. Did I bare my midriff? You betcha, every chance I got. That was then.

In my thirties, I wanted cleavage. In my thirties I could get away with it.

At thirty-five I became a businesswoman and newswoman. But remember, my field was fashion, so I thought I needed glamour, or in this case, bleached blonde hair.

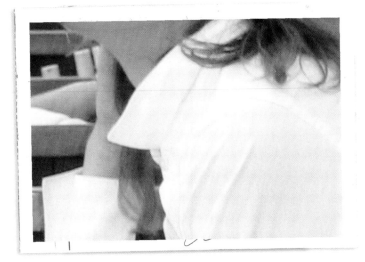

Display your personal style with a mix of updated accessories and individual clothing items: a unique vest, a small fitted jacket, a short cardigan, an unusual belt, layered bracelets, or a bucket hat. Use the trends to your advantage in smaller pieces that mix with your classics, but never overpower them. Think classics 80 percent, trends 20 percent.

As much as I adore the trends and love sharing them with television viewers, I now have to give a disclaimer with my seasonal trend reports. You will hear me say "adapt what is appropriate and mix it in with your existing wardrobe." Trends are made for the very young. Once you know how to distinguish the difference between being too trendy and being totally appropriate, your wardrobe decisions become uncomplicated.

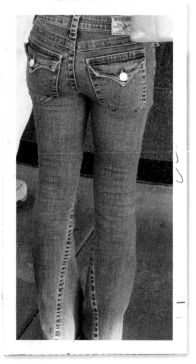

These pockets may be in style but they are far from flattering. Pockets are meant to either hold things or add interest. On our tushes, they do neither.

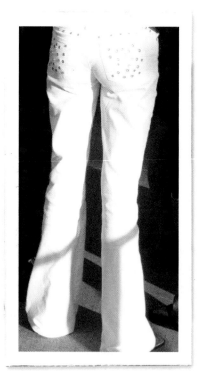

Bright flashing lights would make this gem-decorated tush glow. Is that really what you want your tush to do? Keep the glow in your face and in your heart where it belongs.

FABRIC DISASTERS

Bet you never thought fabrics could get you into trouble, but they can. Many of my friends go to war with me on my views and you can, too, but I promise you they are truths. Here's my fabric insight.

Dating: Not Dinner and a Movie

While we consider most fabrics to be ageless, some can be dating, and I'm not talking dinner and a movie. Your mother might have crocheted that sweater for you, but if it resembles something that decorated her couch, please don't put it on your back. Crocheted or knitted garments that look homemade are cool when you're twenty, but not any more. Avoid wearing anything that resembles a doily.

When I lived in a very suburban area of Los Angeles in the early nineties, everyone over forty wore St. John knits. They became the uniform of the successful. St. John has since changed their styles, but kept their knit fabric. To this day when I see someone in a St. John outfit, even from the back, I know their age.

If you twirled around the dance floor at your prom in layered chiffon you should probably give up both the chiffon and the twirling. The more sheen in your satin, the larger you will look. Shiny is enlarging. Catwoman wears rubber. Madonna wears vinyl at her concerts. Paris Hilton loves metallic. Leave these for them.

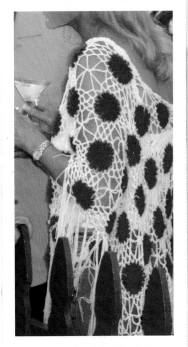

I hope someone made this for her. I wouldn't want to think she spent her money to look like her great aunt's doilies.

Keep the Leather on the Animals

Stop screaming. I know leather is "in." I know style gurus Barbara Walters and Diane Sawyer wear it on television in attractive, buttery pastel shades. I know you probably have several leather items in your closet. Leather has become the "look how cool I am" item for the forty-plus woman. I absolutely, positively disagree. I like leather. I think it looks smart. But it doesn't look soft, even if it feels soft. We look so much better with delicious fabrics by our faces and on our bodies. I know it makes you feel young and hip. It just doesn't make you look it. Honest.

Oprah sometimes wears leather on her talk show. As much as I admire her, I feel she is at her best when she wears magnificent fabrics. But Oprah is Oprah and she can get away with what we mere mortals cannot. Worn by the face, leather is cold and hard, even in the most luxurious quality. Yes, you can add a Pashmina scarf or a handsome, crisp, collar to frame your face, but the leather is still there. It still ages. It's still harsh. It just looks like you're trying too hard.

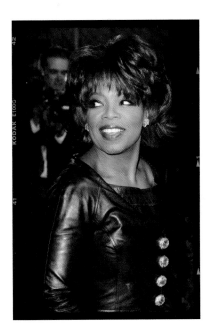

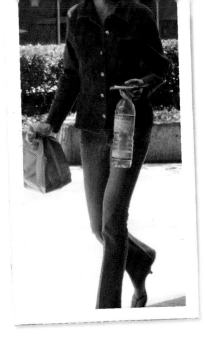

Head-to-toe denim is extreme. We are not about being suited in denim, we are into denim suiting us.

Denimized

I love blue jeans. I love jean jackets. Denim skirts never go out of style. Just don't wear them all together. A little denim is great. Too much denim is dated. Pick one denim item and mix it with cashmeres, luxurious wools, or crisp cottons. Keep your denim pure: no overly frayed hems, layered fringes, decorative studs, or folkloric embroidery.

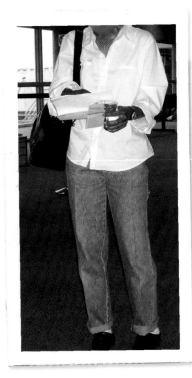

Foolproof dressing: Loose-fitting jeans and a classic white shirt.

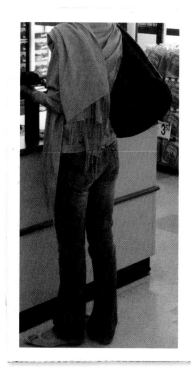

A perfect combination is pairing your favorite jeans with flattering color by your face.

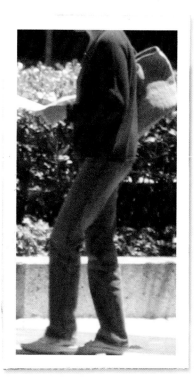

Don't we all love the comfort of jeans and a loose sweater? Accessories take it to the next level.

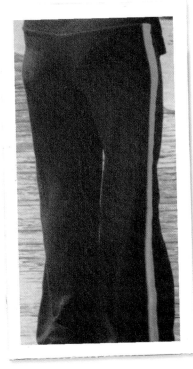

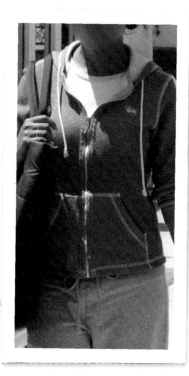

The vertical stripe is supposed to make her look taller, but the fit is making her look lumpier. The solution? One pant size larger and one string thong.

This is the way we want our sweats to look from the rear view: not too baggy, not too tight, just right.

Great sweat style. Mix up your tops and pants so they are not always outfits.

Uniformed Sweats

They are comfy, cozy, and in all the fashion magazines, and yes, we adore them. They have become mainstream dressing, but is that a good thing? Sweats belong at home, in the gym, or perhaps for running errands. I don't feel they should be our costume of choice. Dressing down all the time might suit your lifestyle, but it doesn't suit your style.

A hoodie sweat jacket pairs nicely with jeans or khakis. A pair of sweat pants dresses up a bit with a blazer or sweater. Still, they are sweats. Keep them as a part of your wardrobe, not your uniform.

Revealing your undies is a very sexy, hot trend. If you ever used those tiny gold safety pins to pin your bra straps to your top so they wouldn't show, that's a pretty good indicator that this trend is not for you.

Lingerie is lingerie. Clothing is clothing. A tease of a colorful thong peeping above a waistband is not the kind of teasing we should be doing. A peek of lace on a camisole is romantic as long as it is under a blouse, sweater, or buttoned jacket. Worn alone it says "rock star." Unless you are one, don't do it.

GROWN-UP GIRL'S UNDERWEAR RULE:

Don't let your lace camisoles or tank tops reveal too much.
Have the straps taken up by your tailor so they cover more
chest area. You get the look without the exposure.

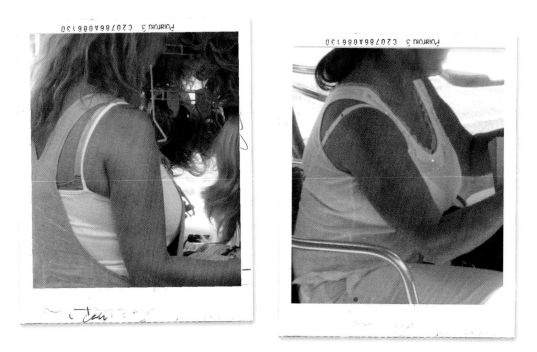

Teens love the look of a revealed bra strap. In their world it's hot. In our world it's bad taste. Teenile is an adjective used to describe someone who is too old for what she is wearing.

Promoting Calvin

What should you do with your Victorian suit, the navy and white yachting sweater, the animal print dress and shoes, and the top with witches and goblins you bring out every Halloween? Donate them to Goodwill.

Themes are good for parks and parties, not for clothing. Don't promote logos, promote yourself. Calvin Klein might want to see his name across your chest; no one else does. Except for trendy teens, who wants Abercrombie on the seat of their pants? Any logo bigger than your pinky finger is too big.

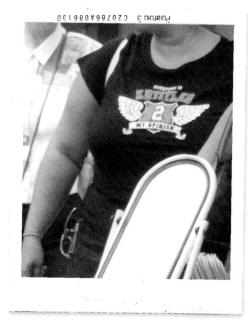

FIT DISASTERS

Body-conscious for fall. Loose and flowing for spring. Baggy for summer. Covered-up and layered for winter. The fit of our fashion changes with the winds in order to keep us shopping. The designers tell us what fit we need and when we need it. They fit the mannequins. We have to fit ourselves. We have real bodies, real curves, and real issues. Most often these don't fit in with the shapes of the moment. The only shape we must be concerned with is our own. Blending the trends with our shape is the challenge.

Oh, for the simplicity and elegance of a solid black, long-sleeve T-shirt.

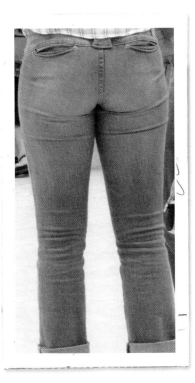

Too much hugging for one pair of jeans to handle. I know we have a love affair with our jeans, but in public?

Hugging Your Butt

Even if you just lost a full dress size, tight is not what you are after. Body-clinging clothing is not flattering. I grant you, a little stretch in fabric makes your clothes comfortable but it also makes them cling. The only thing that should hug your butt is the hand of the one you want. Clothes need to glide over the body. Exercise tights are made for the gym, not the sidewalks. The old "lie on the floor to zip up your jeans" practice is a thing of the past. Don't buy the size you want to be. Buy the size you are or slightly larger. No one will know you have a tiny tummy bulge unless you reveal it. Your ample thighs can be your secret unless you show them.

GROWN-UP GIRL'S TIGHTNESS RULE:

Do a rearview mirror check before you ever leave your house. Is there any unnecessary hugging going on? We always check our front view, but what about the side and back? Everyone else checks these out. Hugging indicates a too tight fit and the need for a little alteration.

Out-of-Style Styles

Love that jacket from the eighties? I guarantee it looks like the eighties. Waiting for padded shoulders to make a comeback? If and when they do, they will be different. The cut and fit of fashion changes. Nothing is more aging than outdated clothes. Don't hang on to out-of-style styles. Renew your favorites. Few items can stand the test of time without major altering. Vintage looks contemporary on the young, on us it just looks old.

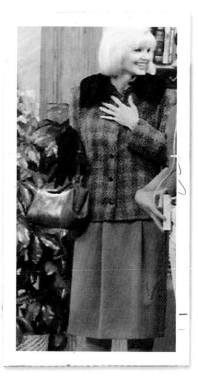

I wore this outfit on a television show in the eighties. Over twenty years later the look is back, however my outfit is not. If I wore this today I would look as vintage as the clothes.

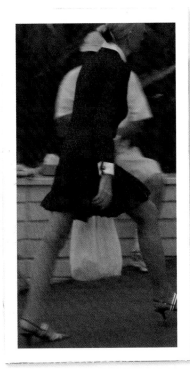

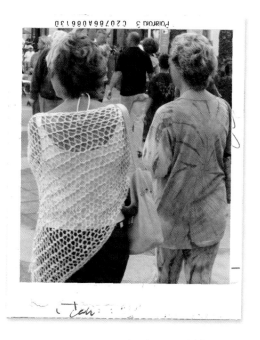

This look is confused. The hair is gray, the hairstyle is mature, the dress is too short, and the shoes are contemporary. Her personal style statement is lost somewhere in the mix.

Friends' influence can either be a good thing or a tie-dye thing. The question is, did they actually buy these outfits or are they leftovers from their '60s Woodstock days?

Shaped Focus

The shape of fashion changes constantly. Nothing is more dated than wearing big jackets when small jackets are in. Fortunately, today we have many choices and as long as you wear those choices in moderation you will look contemporary. It's the extremes that scream "dated." Always consider your figure first, fashion second. If your shoulders are narrow, opt for a small amount of padding in your jackets. If your hips are full, wear loose, fuller cut pants. If your tummy is far from flat, avoid pleats, regardless of what is "in." The compromise is wearing contemporary accessories with your form-flattering classics.

DECORATION DISASTERS

If designers only designed classic clothing they would soon be out of business. It's the frills that keep us wanting what's new—the piping on a jacket, the fringe on a dress hem, the ruffle on a blouse. Every season the frills change. I know, I report them season after season. Frills do create style, but they also create confusion.

How much is too much frill? When you see the trim before you see the person. Chanel has made the fringed jacket a fashion statement but inexpensive copycats have made it an overfringed, unraveling wannabe.

Details are important to your personal style. But they are never important enough to take over your personal statement.

Ruffled and Bowed

We associate ruffles and bows with femininity and romance. Placed by our face, ruffles are soft and flattering. But after forty we not only have to count the pounds and the years, we now have to count our ruffles and bows. A beautiful ruffled collar with one or two layers looks chic peeking out of a tailored jacket or V-neck sweater. A long-sleeved blouse with ruffles at the wrists softens a suit and our hands at the same time. A ruffle around a skirt hem places attention on our legs. Please don't wear them all together. Too many ruffles and we look like we're in *Pirates of the Caribbean*. Pick one place to ruffle or bow at a time. If you love the look of bows on your shoes, that should be your bow allotment for the day. A soft leather or ribbon belt with a bow clasp is sophisticated and feminine. Scarves tied in bows at our neck are matronly. Don't be caught overbowed, and don't mix your ruffles and bows together. We don't want to be cutesy.

Fringes and Trims

I am not a big advocate of fringes and trims. I love the knotted fringe on a pashmina shawl and I like the long gauze fringe on a summer scarf. I have never really liked the fringe on any of the skirts I bought on impulse. I have tired of the jackets with trim on all the seams. The items I reach for over and over are the plainer ones that I can style up. Add a few wonderful accessories to overtrimmed clothes and you have too much going on. Pick your trims in moderation. My home is filled with decorative pillows that are fringed and trimmed to the max. I love them, but I don't have to wear them.

Stitching

Sweaters, jackets, skirts, and pants are considered more stylish with the addition of threads, ribbons, and yarns woven into interesting and creative patterns. They are also more costly. It takes time and talent to add these elaborate accoutrements. But as investments they fall short. A beautiful cardigan with roses embroidered down the side is unique the first time you wear it. But what attracted you to it is what makes it too memorable to wear repeatedly.

The Marilyn Monroe Quick Check

Frilly was not a word associated with Marilyn. She went in for minimalist dressing, sometimes too minimal. She got it right for the image she wanted to project. She also got another thing right. I call it the Marilyn Monroe approach. Each time she left her house she checked her mirror and removed something. Of course it was usually her bra, but I'm talking ruffles, trims, and accessories. The MM quick check can send you out the door accessorized but never overdone.

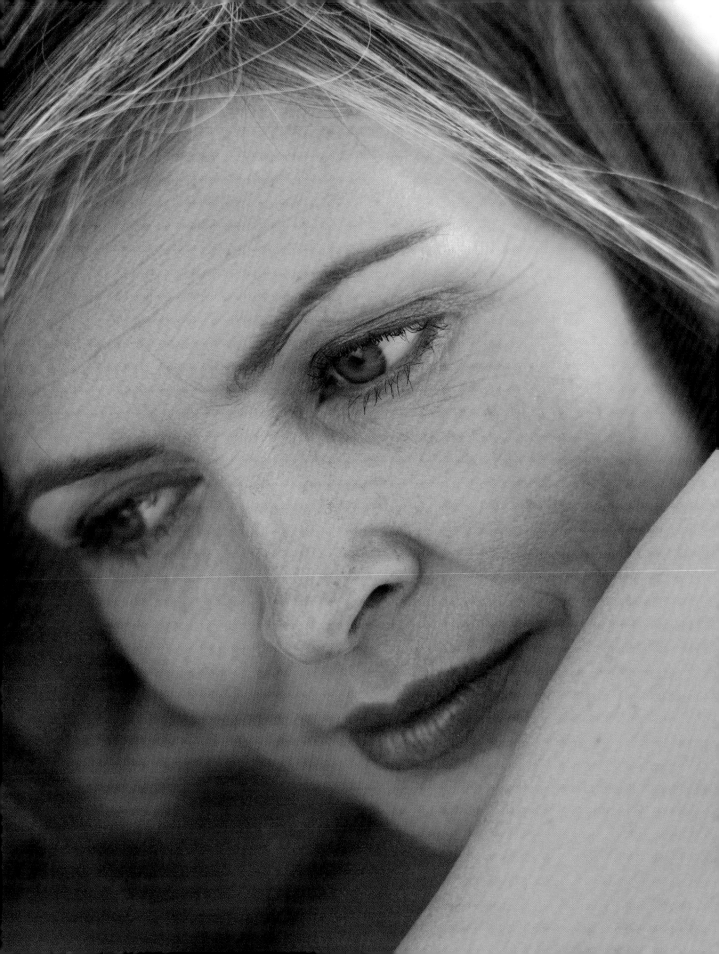

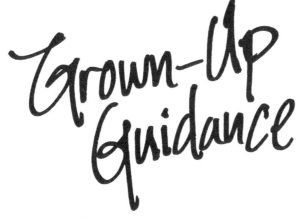

CHAPTER THREE

Grown-Up Guidance

Now that the definition of forty and fifty has changed, we are in need of good role models and they are everywhere. It might be a friend who always looks exquisite or a major celebrity who gets it right. Many leading designers are now addressing the grown-up girl. The Gap is testing merchandise specifically targeted at those over thirty-five in their Fourth & Towne stores. Department stores are allotting more space to the baby boomers. Advertisers are starting to take notice that we are healthy, spending consumers. We are finally getting the attention we deserve.

We need to start at the beginning, and at the beginning is how we see ourselves. See yourself in a positive, ever changing light. I am not recommending you copy Joan Rivers' path of looking forever thirty. I think Joan looks incredibly "perfect" for being over seventy. I just think she has lost the essence of being Joan. What technology you choose to use or not use for maintaining your face and body is a personal decision. When it comes to how you dress your body it's an educated decision. I can't go along with the adage "if it makes you feel good, that's all that matters." I believe if you look good you will feel better. That's where the edification comes in. I am recommending that you open yourself to the possibilities of changes in your style, beauty, and attitude.

Grown-up style is more about what *not* to do. Fashion faux pas become fashion disasters with each passing decade. The more aware we are of the pitfalls, the easier it is to avoid them.

So, what do we do? How do we balance the fashionable with the appropriate? Here are some of my best kept fashion secrets, from the inside out.

Under the Covers

Style starts with your underwear. No one may see it except you, but you will feel it. The right underwear makes everything else you put on look better.

SEDUCTIVELY SECRET

Can you take your clothes off right this very minute and not apologize for your underwear? When you slip into or out of it does it make you feel feminine? Does it feel luxurious against your skin? Does it support you where you need support and hold you in where you need a little impersonal holding?

If you can answer yes to these questions, congratulations! Our undergarments reveal a lot about how we feel about ourselves. They first must enhance our bodies and second make us feel and look seductive, not for anyone other than ourselves. It's that feeling that keeps us smiling in our turtlenecks and longer sleeves.

SCANTY PANTIES

No, no, don't give up your panties; just give up the line that screams "panties." Try some of the new alternatives for a smooth, clean look. Here are my favorite knickers:

The thong *It takes a bit of getting used to. I know, I know, the dental floss joke, but they really work, stick with it.*

Boy shorts or tap pants *Borrowed from men's undergarments, they cover the upper thigh area. Dressed up with a little lace or romantic print, they are sexy and feminine.*

Briefs *Cut high on the leg, they give the best coverage over the tummy and tush areas without looking matronly.*

No-panty line panties *Sorry, but they don't tell the truth. They might not give you the distinctive line of regular panties, but nonetheless, they give you a line. As undergarments, the word that comes to my mind is* boring.

The fuller-proportioned woman omits the panty line by wearing pants and skirts with a looser fit in nonclinging fabrics. Buy full-cut panties in delightful colors, fabrics, and prints with feminine touches of lace and embroidery.

Panties should make you feel good and look good in your clothes. You can be as nice or naughty as you want, or you can use a woman's prerogative and be a little of both.

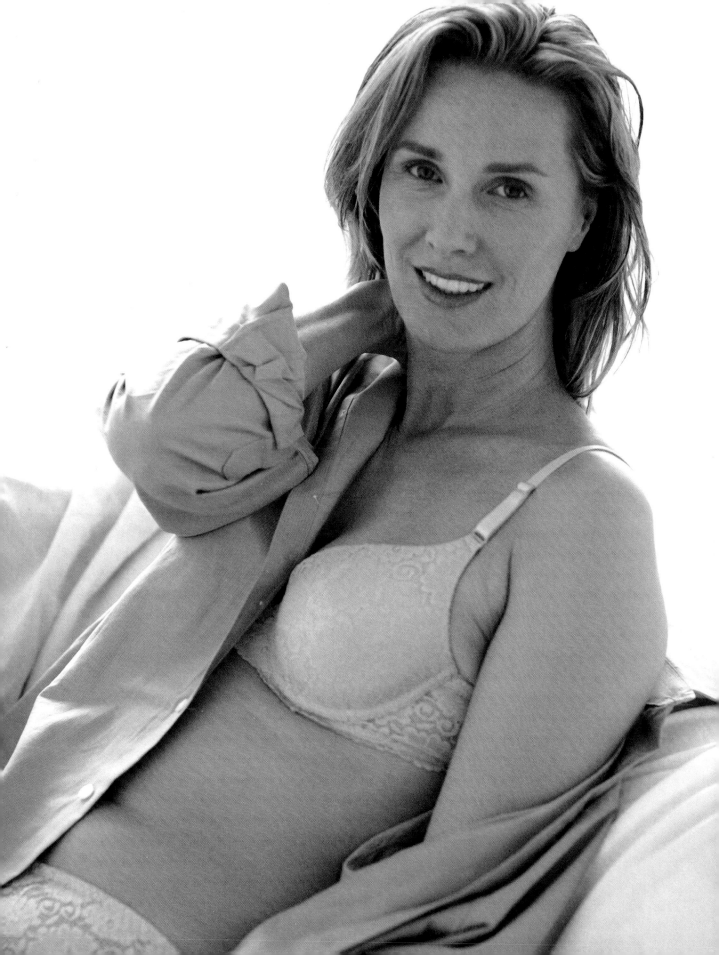

GROWN-UP GIRL'S LINGERIE RULE:

Use lingerie to be as stylish in private as you are in public.

SUPPORT YOUR BOOBS

We're past needing bras to breastfeed or make our nipples perky under T-shirts. We need them to defy gravity. Support is the secret ingredient. Underwires are our best friends. Wider shoulder bands become lifesavers. Are your breasts positioned closer to your shoulder line or your waistline? For the answer, stand sideways and look in the mirror. Mirrors don't lie.

I never did the sideways mirror check. My revelation came as a result of viewing family pictures. Looking through our newly developed Thanksgiving Day photos, there I stood, smiling in my fabulous new pink cashmere sweater, turkey platter in hand. The

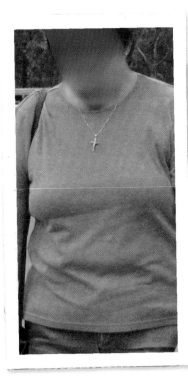 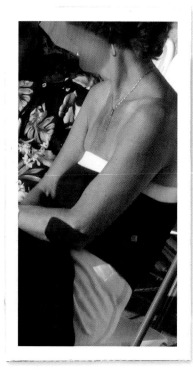 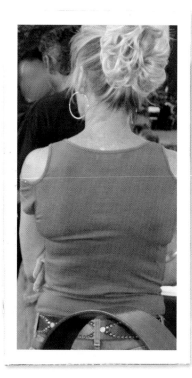

Front views are most obvious. Are your breasts even? Are they in the right position? Are your nipples discreetly covered? Do you look supported without looking fake?

Side views can be the most revealing. Are your breasts closer to your neck or your waist?

We usually forget about the back view, but others don't. Overhang indicates a too tight, ill-fitting bra.

only problem was my boobs (in their feminine, nude color, sheer, barely there bra) were almost on the platter. When had this happened? How is it that I never noticed? Immediately, underwires replaced barely there. Support straps replaced thin silk straps.

Mimi Rogers might have the guts and courage to do full frontal nudity in the movie *The Door in the Floor*, but I heard the gasp of the audience at the sight of her turkey-platter breasts. For the rest of us, support, support, support.

GROWN-UP GIRL'S BRA RULE:

Never leave your house without checking your
bra support from the front, side, and back views.

Bra necessities

Everyday bras should be nude colored, smooth, and seamless. They need to disappear under most garments. Lace makes lumps, so save it for clothing that does not cling.

Sports bras give great comfort and support even if you don't participate in sports. Look for the ones with segregated cups to avoid the flat, pancake look.

Decorative bras come in colors, prints, lace trims, and sheer fabrics. A hint of a white lacy bra under the fabric of a crisp nonclinging shirt can be feminine, but it needs to be only a hint. No cleavage, no nipples, just a whisper of lace. We all need a few decorations, especially on a bad hair day, to keep us sane. Only wear colors and prints under looser tops. We don't need anyone to know we have them on (well, maybe one person).

Minimizer bras reduce breast size by one cup. Their thicker straps and back also give you good support without making indentations in your shoulders. Bras with "wings" also give added support with the extra material along the back and sides.

Posture braces I know it sound dreadful, but are no more dreadful than stooped posture. If osteoporosis is targeting your back, first see your doctor for the latest in medications, then see your medical supply store for a brace that will help keep your shoulders and back straight. Whether you wear it while you sleep or in the comfort of your home, just wear it. Prevention is everything.

Enhancing bras give a little extra boost (no, I didn't say cleavage—remember we are past that). Opt for a bra that has a bump-it-up factor with built-in padding. Stay far, far away from bras that inflate or contain water, silicone adhesives, or gel inserts. Can you even imagine the consequences? Yes, you can get that Pamela Anderson look with a product like Take-Outs inserted in your bra, but why would you want it?

Shop for cotton bras with a small percentage of microfibers for stretch. The addition of spandex-type fabrics helps keep the shape and the fit. Buy the highest quality you can afford and treat it lovingly. Washing by hand is best but many washing machines now have a hand-wash cycle. Never put your delicates in the dryer. Lay them out or hang them up to air-dry. They will last twice as long. On wash day my laundry room looks like a mini-Victoria's Secret store window. I keep a shopping bag on the floor of my closet for my underwear only. This way nothing ends up in the wrong wash pile. Lingerie bags protect the tiniest and laciest of undies during machine wash.

GROWN-UP GIRL'S BRA RULE:
Never show your nipples. Not even a hint.

Save your thin, sheer, barely-there bras for your heavier, thicker tops. Farrah Fawcett boosted the poster business by revealing a hint of nipples under a tight white T-shirt. Her nipples were in their twenties at the time. Someone needs to tell her it's years later. Don't do a Farrah. Cover even the tiniest bit of nipple revelation with a product called Breast Petals. They are floral-shaped, flesh-colored adhesives available in most major department stores. Can't find Petals? Cut the adhesive part of a skin-colored Band Aid (no Sesame Street characters please) and place it over your nipple. This is every fashion stylist's lifesaver on television and movie sets.

Polyfoam Peel-n-Stick Cups give a little more "bare-looking" coverage when Petals won't do the trick. And braless? We may have burned them in the sixties, but today going braless is not even a consideration. The only bounce we should see is the fabric softener in our dryer.

COMPRESSION IS FOR YOUR ZIP FILE

Body sculpting underwear claims to do what to date has only been done with suction and suturing by a plastic surgeon. There is something to hold in almost anything on anybody: thigh shapers, waistline slimmers, belly busters, and butt lifters and separators. Of course you might not be able to sit in comfort, but think how wonderful you'll look standing. Don't delude yourself. Buy them in your size, not the size you want to look. This will enable you to walk and smile at the same time.

Does this give you permission to wear tight, tight, tight? NO! Tight only looks squeezed in with these magical items. They only work under looser clothing. If you wear them under your size 6 jeans when you are a size 10, the whole world will know what you are doing. Knits and silks will still cling; the weight will still be there. Who wants a flat, squeezed-looking tush?

Under your more body-conscious clothes, stick with basic control pantyhose. Tummy control, hip and thigh controls, and butt lifts make this the choice for slimming. They give us a smoother, cleaner line without the compressed look of heavier under-garments. Just make sure you buy pantyhose with a cotton crotch because you never, ever want to wear your undies with your pantyhose.

On Top of the Covers

Once you have the underwear necessities covered, literally, it's time to concentrate on what you put over them. Just walk through any mall and you can't help but be over-whelmed by the variety of clothing stores. Too many fashionable choices? My guide-lines will help you focus on what really works and what doesn't.

DESIGNER DIGS

GROWN-UP GIRL'S DESIGN RULE:

Borrow from the designers.

Well, not actually. Fashion designers only lend to celebrities like Catherine Zeta-Jones and Nicole Kidman, but you can visit their boutiques or designer sections in the department stores. It doesn't cost anything to look. Donna Karan and Calvin Klein might present risqué on the runway, but on the racks they understand the brilliant bal-ance between bare and there.

Karan knows the importance of covering arms with her shrugs and long-sleeved tops. Because she knows most shoulders and backs are firm and bony, she chooses to reveal these areas with seductive geometric-shaped cutouts. Klein continues to include midknee skirts and dresses in his line. They know the value of what to reveal and what to cover. They also know who their buyers are: upper-crust women with money to spend.

GROWN-UP GIRL'S BUYING RULE:

Expand your wardrobe by buying more tops than bottoms.

What is the size range on the clothes in your closet? My guess is between two and three sizes, depending on the designer and brand. In J.Crew and Banana Republic I wear a size 6 or 8. In Ralph Lauren I wear a size 4. Because I am paying more, all of a sudden I'm smaller? Who doesn't like to see a small size when they step into their pants? It's called vanity sizing and it's great marketing.

Size does not matter! If you are wearing your size on the back of your jeans for the public to see, shame on you! Fit matters. When in doubt, buy one size larger and alter. Pants should fall straight. They must fit in the rear. Pockets need to lie flat or be removed. Jackets should ease over your shape. Skirts should glide, not hug your body. Most cleaners have in-house tailors and now is the perfect time to make their acquaintance. The money you spend on tailoring is an important investment in yourself.

THE COLOR DIET

"Lime green is the 'in' color for spring. Brown is the new black. Purple and red are the hot combo. Think pink!" Have you heard these before? You probably have heard them from me when I do a trend segment on a television talk show. It's my job to report the latest and unfortunately there is never time to place caveats where they belong.

Color can be your best asset or your worst enemy. Too much color will overpower. Small amounts of color will enhance. Choose your colors wisely, place them on your body appropriately, and wear them sparingly. Let me break it down for you.

- *The neutrals* should make up the majority of your wardrobe. Black, white, navy, gray, and earth colors are your building blocks. Choose neutral over a brightly colored suit. Yes, Laura Bush and Hillary Clinton do wear turquoise suits. Their goal is to attract a crowd, stand out on television, and be the center of attention. Unless you are a politician, a talk show host, or a public speaker, neutrals will always serve you best.

- *Complimentary colors* are the ones that gather you the most compliments and are the most important colors to keep by your face. "You look wonderful in powder pink." "You look extraordinary—what did you do differently?" you hear when you wear a robin's egg blue sweater; "Your skin looks radiant" when you wear your butter yellow scarf. These are the colors that complement your skin tone. Build a wardrobe of scarves, sweaters, shirts, jackets, hats, earrings, and necklaces in these colors. The colors you wear next to your face should flatter you. The colors you wear on your body can work for you if you choose properly.

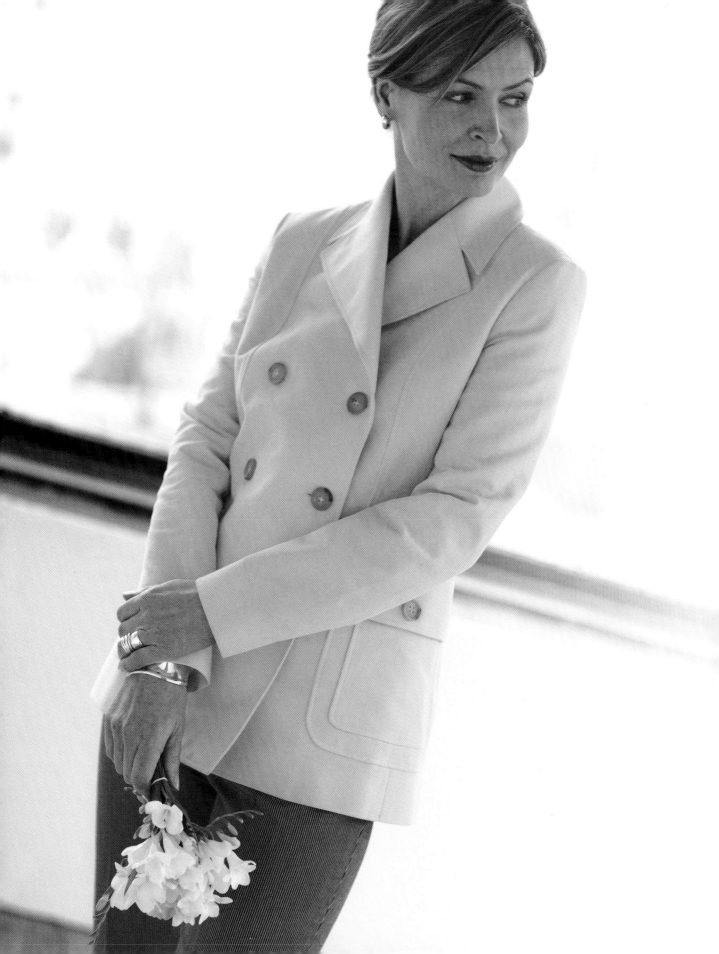

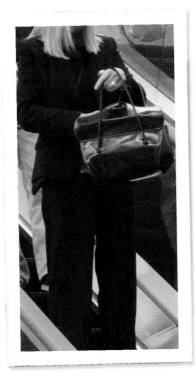

Head-to-toe black will always make you look taller, slimmer, and smarter. There's a reason we fill our closets with the kindest of colors.

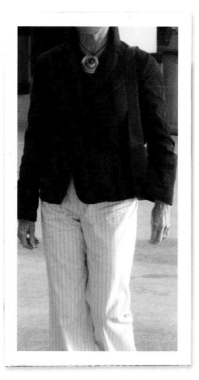

Neutral perfection. Classic and elegant with a large accessory twist.

- *Accent colors* are the bold or electric brights you add in the mix. A scarlet red dress gathers attention. A canary yellow sweater can lift your spirits. A periwinkle blue jacket might be calming. A good rule to follow is: the brighter the color the less of it you wear. If lime is your favorite color, opt for a scarf, top, or accessory.

- *Muddy colors* are colors that are subdued with gray. The overall effect is mucky. Grayed wines, blues, and browns may look nice in your draperies or on a sofa, but by your face they are simply dull. Who needs dull when there are so many flattering colors?

- *Diet colors* are the dark colors that slim. If you want to look and feel ten pounds lighter, put on black, charcoal, navy, or chocolate brown. The darker the color, the slimmer you will look. The lighter or brighter the color the larger you will appear.

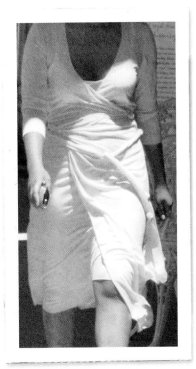

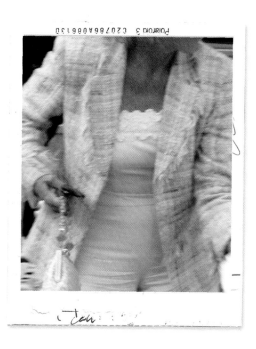

Walking toward us is a lime green dress. We never want to be identified by our dress color; we want to be identified by our style.

This grown-up girl uses two basic fashion guidelines to her advantage:

1. Wear beautiful colors and collars by the face.

2. When you have a jacket in one color, keep what you wear under it in the same second color from top to bottom.

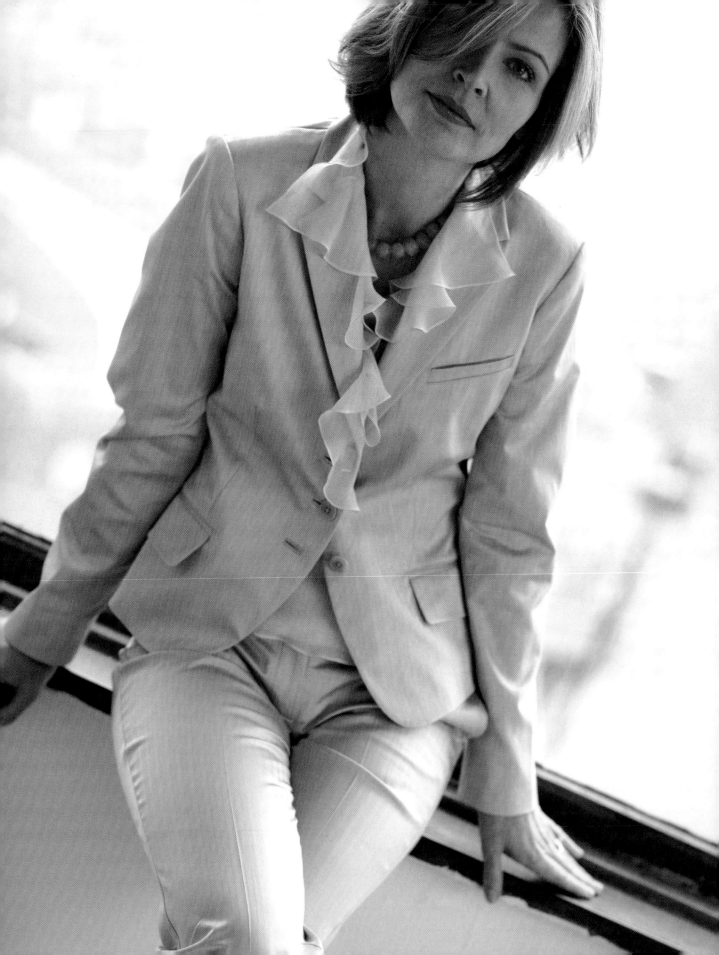

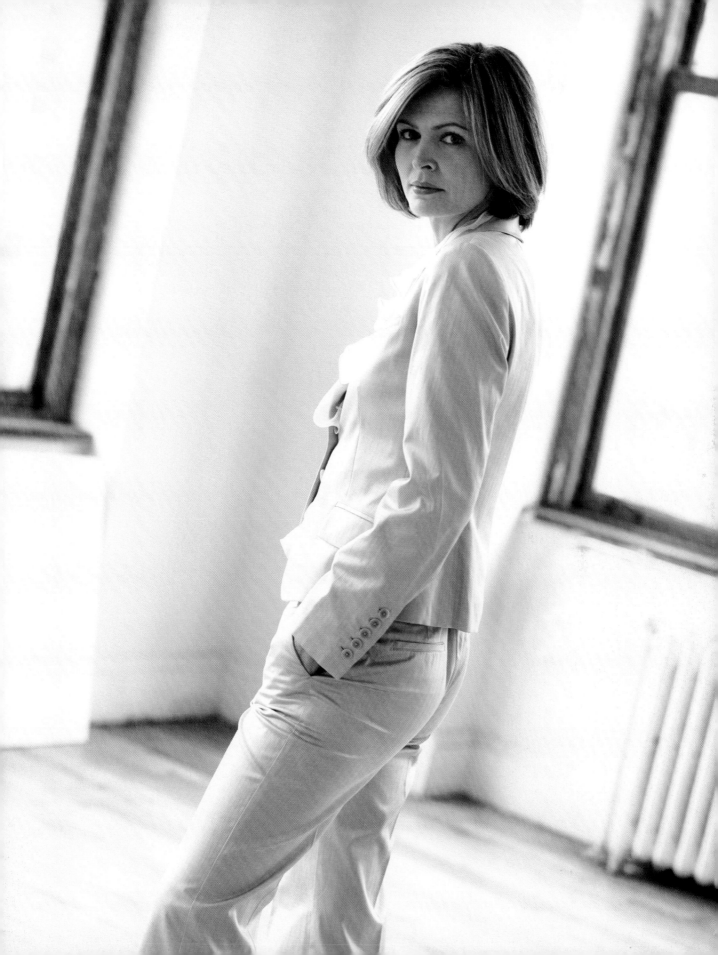

No matter how beautiful the print, how expensive the fabric, or how prominent the designer, you will always look better in solids.

This doesn't mean you can't wear prints, just keep them smaller and as an accent. As we develop a few lines, gain a few pounds, and perhaps add a pair of reading glasses, we need to simplify. Mix this with prints and we have high-wattage dressing.

Pucci might be making a comeback, but we are moving forward. Burberry is building an empire on their trademark plaid but I say wear it in a scarf or just on the cuffs of a coat. Wild animal prints are a signature of Versace, but they shouldn't be yours. You are creating your own individual image, not theirs.

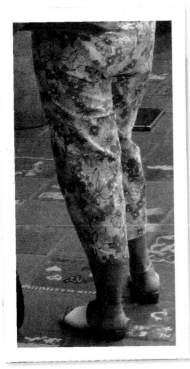 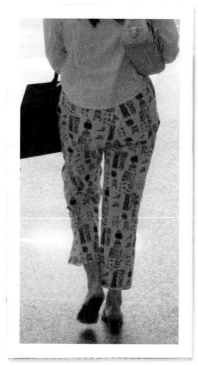 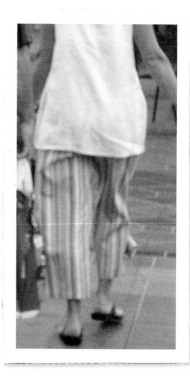

There really isn't a floral print small enough to wear in a pant unless you are size 2. Can anyone's hips really afford flowers?

A man-tailored small stripe in a slightly fuller cut would have been a better choice if a print pant was essential.

If you are yearning for a print, this soft vertical stripe does the job. It elongates and slims the figure.

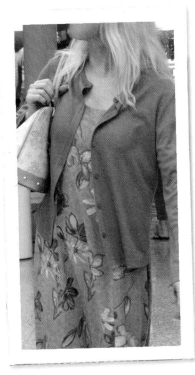

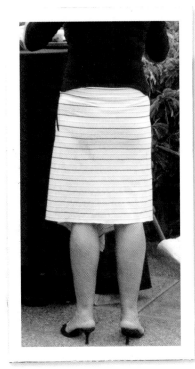

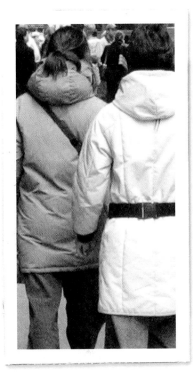

If you love prints, style them up with a solid color sweater, scarf, or jacket by your face. The solid color frames your face. The busy print fights for attention. Who needs the fight?

We have all read and heard that horizontal lines widen. Do we ever want to widen our tushes?

Puffy quilting looks better on beds than on our backs. They may be warm, but they're big.

BULKING UP

Simplicity. I have to say it again, because unless you are into the minimalistic dressing of Calvin Klein, today's styles have more complexity. Complexity adds bulk. A decorative pocket, layering T-shirts and tanks under everything, shirttails hanging out untucked under sweaters, and belted jackets all add bulk. We can do many of these things only if we are aware of their placement.

The popular cargo pant is now a wardrobe basic, but oh, those pockets can get you into trouble. If you are wild for cargo pants, buy them and wear them with traditional items. First check out where the pockets lie. Pockets add bulk, so make sure they are in the slimmest areas. Who needs bulk on their butt, padding on their thighs, or pouches on their tummies?

Layering makes clothing look more interesting, the secret comes in using light layers. Start with the thinnest T-shirt possible for the first layer, a blouse without pockets or gathers for the second, then a lightweight sweater for the third, and finally an unadorned, flat fabric jacket for the fourth. Style up without bulking up.

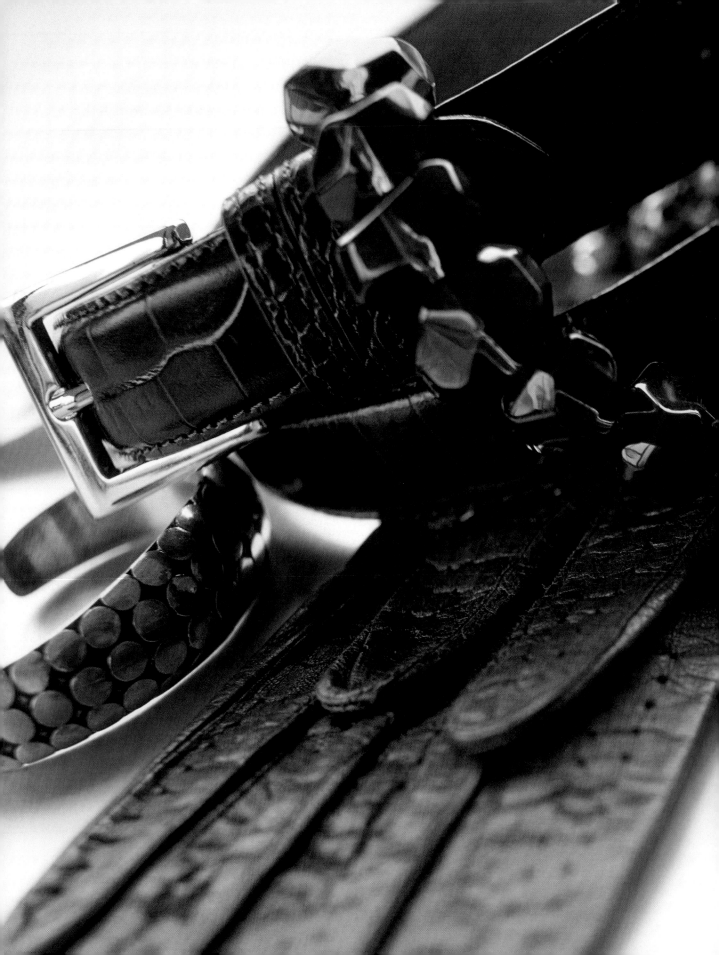

CHAPTER FOUR

The "A" Word: The Grown-Up Girl's Style Secret

"A" stands for accessories. As we pare down our clothing trends, accessories take over as our single most important fashion element. Whimsical, ethnic, vintage, romantic, tailored, sporty, even trendy accessories now create our style. Accessorizing is the most irresistible element of dressing. It can also be the most defining in both the positive and the negative sense.

Never throw out an accessory. The fabric flowers you wore in the eighties made a comeback in 2000. Chanel's characteristic piled-on, layered pearls and textured chains never went out of style. A good belt is a good belt. A pin changes style depending on where you place it. Bracelets take on different looks depending on what you layer together. Old watches are now stylishly vintage. Unlike clothing that changes in silhouette year after year, accessories remain forever. Let's take a detailed look at our new secret weapons.

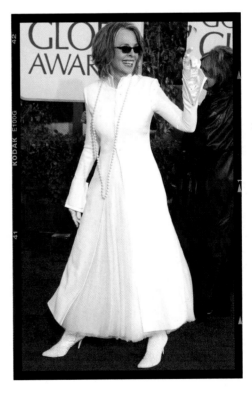

In my book Diane Keaton is the accessory queen. She mixes the elegant, sweet, and bold together and creates her own distinctive look.

Shoe Fetish

How do we combine style and comfort? No one looks good with a pained expression on their face as they try to walk in three-inch Jimmy Choos. On the other hand, no one looks good in orthopedic shoes, even with a smile. There is no reason to give up comfort for style or vice versa. There are plenty of options.

Remember, you don't have to wear the trends, you just have to wear good quality and design. I would rather see you own three basic pairs of delicious shoes than twenty pairs of gimmicky ones. Quality always shows; it also feels comfortable and treats your tootsies with the respect they deserve. Forget that pointed toes are in. Forget rounded toes are back. Forget that stilettos are "hot." What you need are good shoes with style. Just as there are no definite styles in fashion, shoes have followed suit. Round toes, square toes, pointed toes, low heels, high heels, or rubber heels, the choice is yours.

Follow these guidelines:

Loafers. These classics are the perfect companion to pants and many skirts. The newer styles have thicker, flexible soles that are both cushioning and good looking.

Sneakers are style setters. You don't need home court advantage to own several pairs. When your feet hurt, they provide comfort. Big enough to accommodate shoe pads or orthotics, they support you in style. Don't go too far into the retro or futuristic styles. Extremes will be out of style by the time you break them in.

Wearing khakis with a chocolate brown turtleneck? Add a brown and orange sneaker. Cool! Colorful sneakers style up your neutral colored outfits.

Sandals require two important tests before you wear them in public. First, do your feet look good? Feet are not the best part of anyone's anatomy, so it is imperative that you examine yours closely. Second, are they well-groomed? Are your heels soft and your toes nicely polished? If you can answer yes to these questions you are sandal-worthy. If not, try one of the other options.

Lace-up oxfords finish off a tailored menswear look. Try adding a white or masculine print sock.

Pumps. Even a 1-inch pump will make you appear taller and slimmer. Sling backs are fine if your heels are soft and attractive. A peekaboo toe is sexy if those toes are worthy and well-groomed. Otherwise, cover, cover, cover.

Pair a pump in a solid color with a neutral-colored outfit. A navy pantsuit with lime-green shoes. Focusing on only one color is sophisticated.

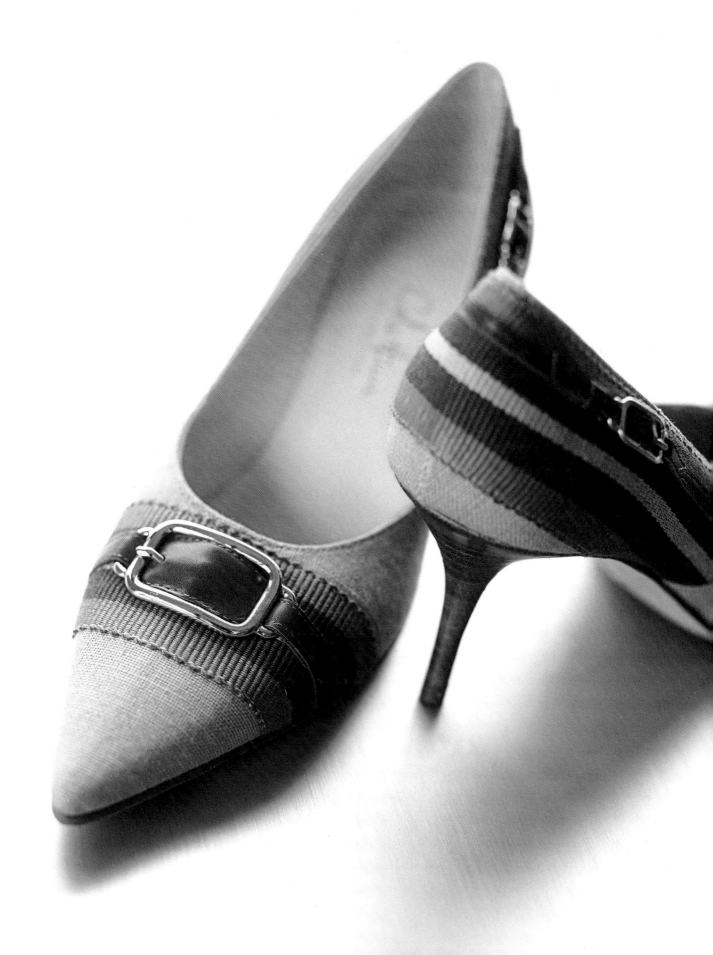

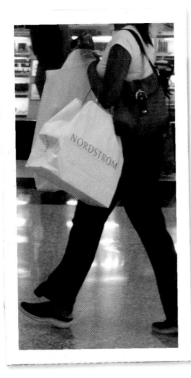

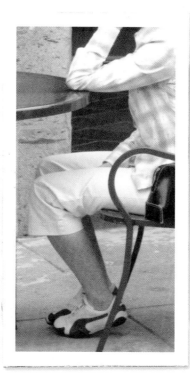

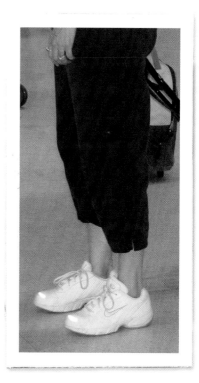

These whimsical, backless sneakers reveal a sense of style, confidence, and independence by not matching the bag to the shoes.

Sometimes it only takes one item to show that you have style. In this classic casual outfit the contemporary sneakers make her fashion statement.

Anything that even resembles a real gym shoe should stay in the gym.

Printed pumps *in bold florals, rich brocades, or whimsical stripes and dots can punch up a classic, neutral-colored outfit. Just don't mix them with clothes of the same pattern. Matching is not only not important, it's outdated.*

For evening, try a closed pump in black or the darker metallics like bronze or pewter. *Leave the gold and silver shoes for Cinderella, the clear plastics for Barbie dolls, and the rhinestone-decorated sandals for the generation Xers. We want our sparkle by our face, not our feet.*

Boots cover a lot of territory. *Flat or heeled, just keep them on the plainer side. If you don't ride a Harley, don't wear motorcycle boots. Fitted to the knee, ankle or cropped boots go best with pants. Knee-highs work with skirts or dresses. Leave the thigh-highs in the store.*

Pamper your feet with shoe pads. Dr. Scholl's has been in business a long time for a good reason. Take the stress off the pad of your foot and protect your heels. Whatever your needs, the doc has a solution for you.

If you have severe foot problems, invest in custom-made orthotics from a podiatrist. They make a mold of your foot and design a shoe pad that fits your specific requirements. Remove the original shoe pads in sneakers, oxfords, or boots and insert your own for instant relief.

GROWN-UP GIRL'S SHOE RULE

Contemporary shoes elevate you to a new level of style.

Shoe Tips

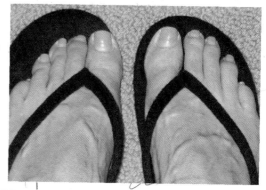

- Don't expose a foot that has broken veins, calluses, bunions, or squished or twisted toes. Leave the sandals on the shelf and buy a covered shoe. Remember, it's not how great the shoes are, it's how great they look on *your* feet.

- If you do reveal your heels or toes, keep them well groomed. Foot grooming says a lot about body grooming. Are you giving the right message?

- Don't match your shoes to your outfit. We are thankfully past uniforms.

These flip-flops might be cool but ready for prime time? Not on these feet!

- Never wear any heel higher than those in which you can walk gracefully. Wobble is not the gait we want.

- Ankle straps, ankle wraps, or T-straps put the focus on your ankles. Are they slim enough to warrant focus?

- Flip-flops might be cool and comfy, but they should not leave your house on a regular basis.

Glam Gams

The legwear section of department stores keeps expanding, giving us way too many options. You need a guide just to decipher it all.

- Determine the density of your stockings by the skin on your legs. The better your skin texture, the sheerer the stockings.

- Try tummy, thigh, control pantyhose: They hold you in, firm you up, and with a cotton crotch, replace panties and panty lines.

- Wear semiopaque or opaques in dark colors if your legs are less than perfect. They cover, slim you down, and create a taller appearance if you dress in a dark neutral color from head to toe.

- Give patterns a try with pants. In subdued, small, tailored prints they add panache to demure, solid color, or monochromatic outfits.

Spray-on or rub-on nylon products like Prescriptives Magic, Air Stockings, or Sally Hanson Airbrush Legs look good in photographs, but in real life the look depends on the application. If you are good with artificial tanning products, give these a try. They can blend your brown spots and dots, making them less noticeable. Just like self-tanners, go for just a little color. If application is not your talent, go for the real deal or go nude, just don't go liquid.

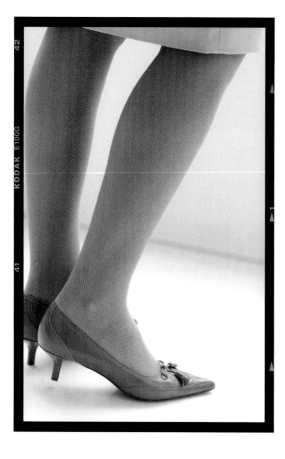

Add a touch of sex appeal with small patterned fishnets. I adore them. Nude-colored fishnets are impossibly elegant under skirts. Black or chocolate brown fishnets are delightful with matching color skirts or pants. The caveat is to keep your skirts on the longer side; a little fishnet goes a long way. If your legs need more coverage (as even our model's did) a pair of nude pantyhose under your fishnets will give you extra coverage.

Recently I was shopping when, ahead of me, I noticed a great pair of legs in a very short pleated skirt, nude fishnet hose, and stiletto pumps. She looked fabulous . . . until she turned around. Her face didn't match her body. Her face was fifty, her body was thirty. Even with great legs, the imbalance was too far off the charts to work. Instead, her legs worked against her.

- Don't invest in shiny stockings. They make legs look larger and bring attention to veins, bruises, or sunspots.

- Don't get your tan from stockings. Tan stockings only work if your body is tanned and I hope for your sake it's not. Tan legs will look like they belong on another body.

- Refuse to buy white, pastel, or brightly colored stockings. White is perfect for nurses, pastels look good on our daughters or granddaughters, and brights—who wants red or turquoise legs? Try a bone color if you need another option.

- Never wear nude-colored support nylons with skirts. Try as they might, they still look like you need a prescription to buy them. If you need support with skirts go to a dark color. If they don't work with your light colors or summer clothes, forgo skirts and wear pants.

- Avoid sparkling or decorated stockings with skirts for dressy evenings. Just like shoes, we don't want our bling bling that low on our bodies. Now, on our ears, that's another story.

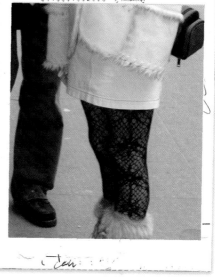

Remember the key word with patterns is small. Does she really think that her legs are looking hot on this cold winter day?

Park Avenue in Des Moines

Socks can add a touch of panache peaking out from under pants or jeans. They can also be utilitarian. Perish the thought! All right, you need those little ankle socks for your tennis shoes when you actually wear them for sports, but short of track, field, or court, make sure they are chic.

Knee-highs give us the look without the restraint of full pantyhose. Just keep your knee-highs under pants. I don't know of a skirt that is long enough to guarantee it won't blow up or move up as you cross your legs. Does Grandma Gurdy come to mind? Knee-highs must never, ever be worn with skirts or dresses. No exceptions!

Small patterned or colored socks give an edge to classic outfits. If you are an individualist, try a bright red, hunter green, or passionate purple pair of socks as long as everything else about your outfit is subtle.

White cotton or cashmere socks and loafers with trousers say "Park Avenue society," even in Des Moines.

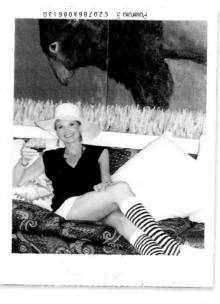

Restraint was not a word I used in my twenties. If a little stripe was good, how could a lot of stripe be bad?

A Bentley on Your Arm

Handbags are the new status symbols. The Hermes Kelly bag is now seen on everyone from twenty to seventy, in all materials from crocodile to rubber, at all price ranges, and in a variety of locations from street vendors to boutiques. We can't seem to get enough of designer bags. Like the cars we drive, the bag we carry defines us, or so we are told. Who wants a Volkswagen when there are such great, affordable knockoffs that we can all have Bentleys?

You need a handbag wardrobe to cover all your requirements:

- **Daytime bags** Your daytime bag should be practical. It has to hold what you must carry without putting your back into spasm. It needs to be large enough not to bulge and small enough to be manageable. I am not a big fan of changing bags daily. I prefer one or two good quality, natural leather bags to get me through a season.

- **Totes** This is a larger, open style bag that carries everything from magazines to water bottles. Keep it in the same color range as your bag. Be nice to your back and pack light.

- **Fanny packs** Don't discount this little treasure. It may not be on the bestseller list, but you can still find them in catalogs, on the Web, in travel stores, and many luggage shops. This is the bag of choice when you need your hands free. Perfect for traveling, shopping, hiking, or babysitting, it allows you to carry your necessities around your waist in comfort. Keep it in solid, neutral leather or nylon fabric. Don't buy one that says "Disneyworld." Wear it slightly looser on your waist. This is not a waist cincher. This is our backpack replacement.

- **Backpacks** Backpacks are fashionable and practical, but not for the grown-up girl. Our backs don't need any additional weight. Just read the posture section (pages 202–4) and you will pack your backpack away.

- **Evening bags** Whereas our evening shoes need to be on the conservative side, we can make up for it with our evening purses. Whimsical, vintage, print, glittering, or glamorous small bags add just the right touch to dressy attire.

- **Colored leather bags** Here's one delicious trend that you can adapt. Citrus yellow, kiwi green, or blush pink, candy-colored bags add casual chic. Don't match them to anything. Buy only good quality leather. No rubber or plastics, please!

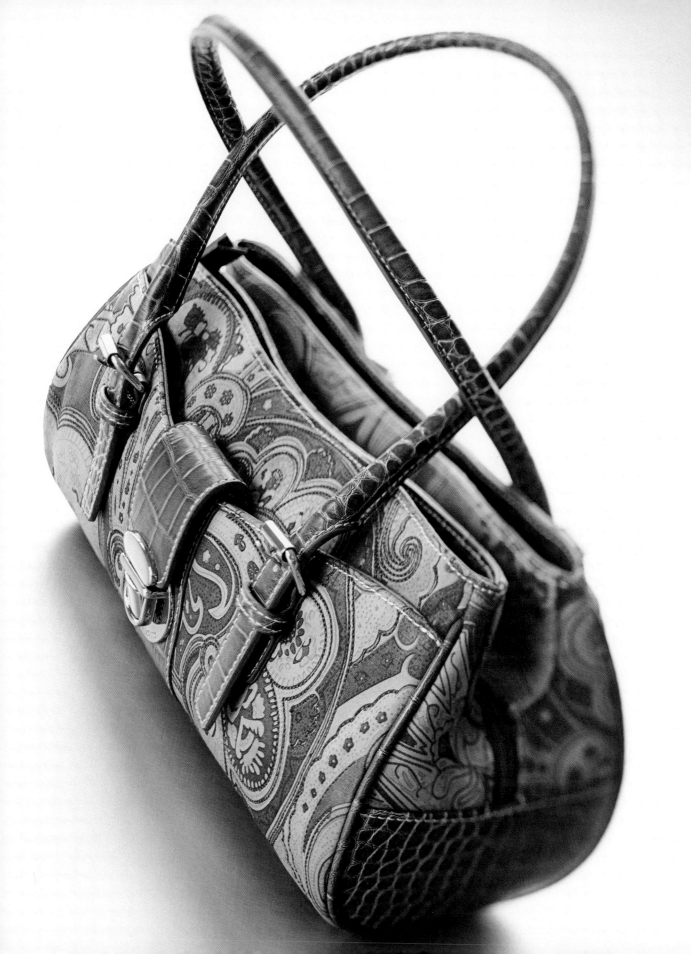

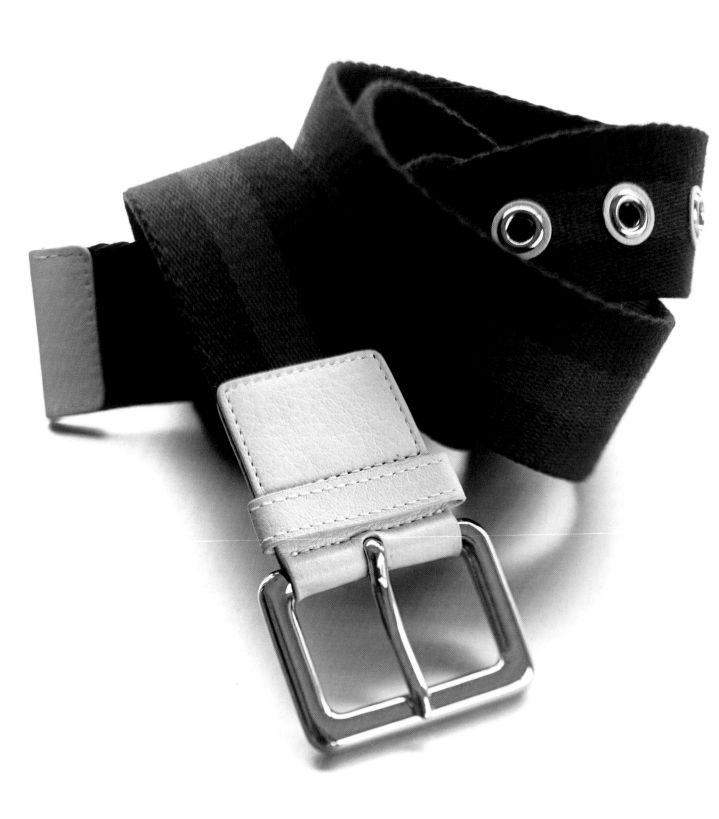

The Horizontal Slash

Belts are made for small waistlines. Who needs to belt in a large waist? Why make a horizontal slash in the middle of your body? The smaller your waist, the more interesting and detailed the belt can be. A pink, lavender, and blue ribbon belt dresses up blue jeans. A silver-buckled brown crocodile belt enriches a black turtleneck and pants. A red leather belt punches up an all gray outfit. *Only use belts on a small waist!* On a large waist it screams "look at my waist size." Do you really want to do that?

Low-slung hip belts give a sensual suggestion, *if* you have small hips. Otherwise you might as well wrap a cloth tape measure around your hipline. Remember, belts emphasize tummies, so keep them on the looser side. A belt is not a corset, go up a belt hole or a size, whatever it takes to make the belt fit with ease.

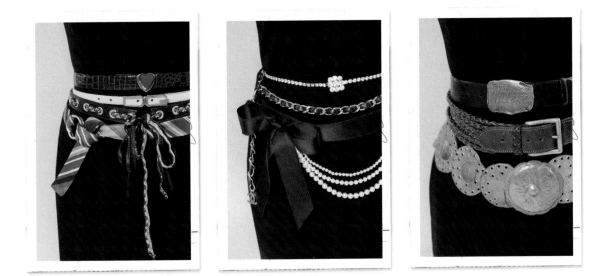

No, don't wear this many at a time. Colorful, evening, or decorative leather belts—own a few of each if your waist is belt-worthy.

Necking

Our necks are one of the first things to exhibit aging. Examine your neck mercilessly: first in a magnifying mirror and second in your car makeup or rearview mirror. Do both in broad daylight; no soft lighting for us, we want the truth. Jack Nicholson might have told Tom Cruise "You can't handle the truth," in the movie *A Few Good Men*. But we are a few good women and we can. Turn your head side to side. If your neck is firm and taunt, skip this section. If it looks dehydrated, go to the chapter on skin. If it looks wrinkled, cover it.

Simply, *don't show what you don't want seen.*

THERE ARE THREE WAYS TO CAMOUFLAGE YOUR NECK EFFECTIVELY

1. Collars

A beautiful collar not only covers your neck, it also enhances your face. A little eyelet trim, a delicate scallop, a touch of embroidery, or a hint of color can be the perfect frame for your face. Add collars under sweaters, jackets, or vests. Turn lightly starched collars up for additional framing. Place a beautiful pin to hold the collar in place. The shorter your hair, the more important collars are to your appearance. They fill in the neck area with interest and softness.

2. Jewelry

Necklaces, boleros, and chokers also do the job if they cover the areas of the neck that need covering. Remember, they must cover, otherwise they draw the eye to areas where we don't want the extra attention. They should be wide without being tight. Tight works when you look head-on but has a tendency to wrinkle the skin as you move from side to side. Can we keep our heads straight when we talk? I doubt it. See the Jewels and Gems section (page 81) for more about jewelry.

3. Scarves

Next to a turtleneck, nothing covers a neck better than a scarf. Any solid-colored scarf wrapped or tied around your neck covers, adds color to your face, and enhances your outfit. This is multitasking at its best. Remember prints are eye-catching, but also distracting when you really want all eyes on you.

The closer to your face you wear the scarf, the better. The style of wrapping extra-long oblong scarves around your neck is perfect for creating style, lengthening the torso with a vertical line, and covering the neck.

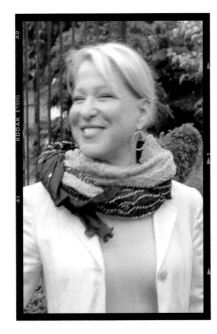

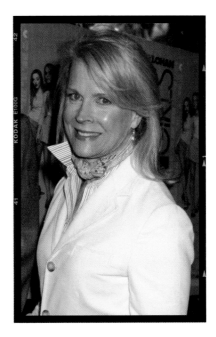

Bette Midler knows that if one scarf is good, two can be better. They frame, flatter, and are simply fantastic.

Candice Bergen uses small scarves as chokers. The style secret is in making the square knot in the front. Roll your scarves on the bias and tie the square knot in the middle.

A good scarf is the next best thing to good makeup. In the right color, it illuminates your skin tone, enhances your eye color, and complements your hair. You need a complete wardrobe of solid color wool, cotton, and silk scarves in a variety of sizes and shapes.

GROWN-UP GIRL'S SCARF RULE

Never throw a scarf out unless it is stained or damaged.

Balance all your neck coverings with a little roll-up or slight push-up of your long sleeves to reveal just a bit of arm. We don't want to walk around looking like mummies, wrapped from head to toe.

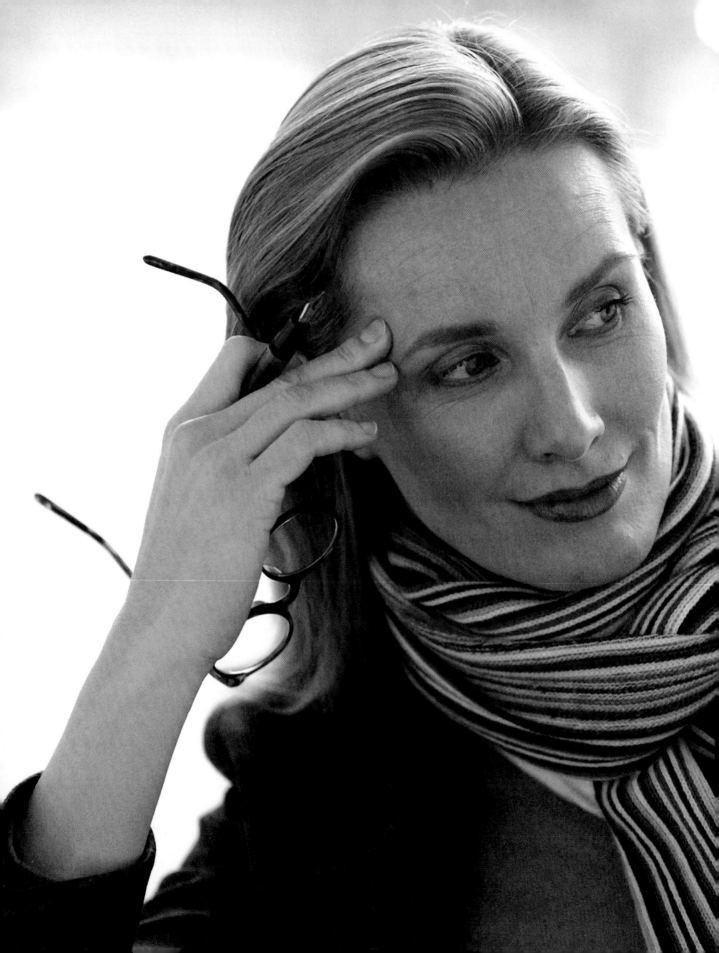

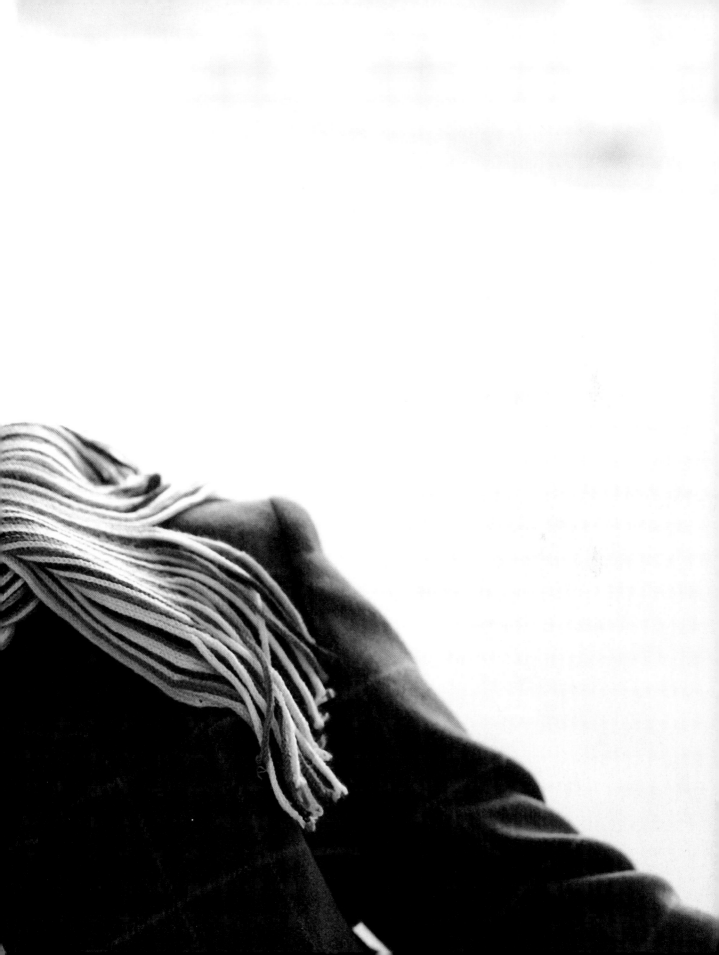

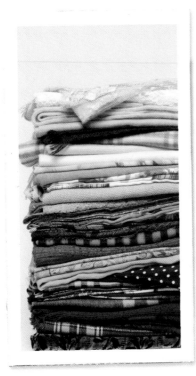

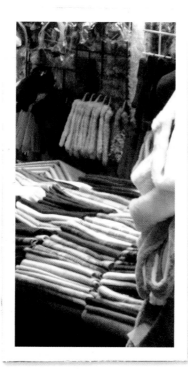

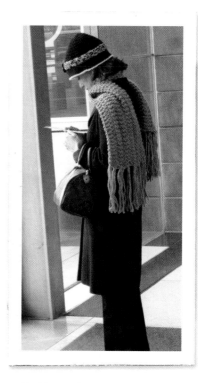

My scarf wardrobe. Some old, some new, all priceless.

Incredible prices, amazing choices. I know major style gurus who buy many of their scarves from street vendors.

Nothing perks up a winter coat— and your spirits—as much as a colorful scarf.

The Breeding Touch

Gloves have made a tremendous comeback. Once reserved for society and cold weather, they are now stylishly chic. This is a trend we can adopt because it works in two ways. First, gloves cover our hands in style and color. Forty-plus years of use can take a toll, so covering is sometimes a good thing. Second, they make you look and feel elegant.

Colorful wools and leathers brighten our basic coats. This is one area where you can match your gloves to your scarf or knit hat. Just don't match all three. Overmatching is just too kitschy. Cotton and lace gloves flatter summer dresses and suits.

A very "Vogue" look with gloves is to push the sleeves of your suit jacket up just below the elbow and wear elbow gloves scrunched down so the jacket and the glove meet. Evening gloves recall glamour and good breeding. Just remember to remove them when you eat.

GROWN-UP GIRL'S JEWELRY RULE:

Check all jewelry for the "wrinkle factor." Abandon anything that causes droop, creases, or wrinkles in your outfit or on your body.

Jewels and Gems

Nothing defines a stylish woman more than her jewelry. I like the idea of combining jewelry styles. Mix the good stuff with the fun stuff; not everything has to be Tiffany. Today, costume jewelry is affordable and fabulous. I mix an antique-etched silver cuff with three bold, black, plastic bracelets. I may combine my Cartier gold tank watch with a gold mini heart bracelet and ten thin elastic bands of white, silver, and bronze beads. Who can tell a diamond from a cubic zirconium tennis bracelet? It's not what you pay, it's how you put it together. Matching jewelry sets are out, and eclectic, distinctive mixing is in.

STICKLERS

Pins are a brilliant method of decorating your clothing. A large antique brooch on a jacket, a cluster of insects or animals, fabric flowers, rhinestone initials, groupings of stickpins, or playful plastic shapes; pins allow you to create your own visual feast.

Place them at the neckline of a blouse, the shoulder of a blazer, the sleeve of a sweater, or the buckle of a belt or purse. Bunch them together on a lapel of a jacket by color, metals, or themes. Never throw a pin out. They are timeless.

I nail a 3-inch wide by 6-foot long piece of black grosgrain ribbon on my closet wall and pin all my pins and flowers to it. This enables me to easily see what I have when I am putting my outfits together.

HAND DÉCOR

Rings decorate your hands. When you took inventory of your body, did your hands pass muster? If so, rings are wonderful. If not, they draw attention we don't need. If you yearn for diamonds, place them by your face, not on your fingers. The only exception is wedding or sentimental keepsakes. If you have beautiful hands, by all means add brazen, over-the-top or layered rings.

Today, watches are considered as much a style accessory as a necessity for telling time. Collect watches and change them with your mood. There are so many affordable watches that you can invest in several. Try changing your watchbands. A bright golden yellow watchband says "creative." Try a bold red band next month, a delicate baby blue after that. It's like having a brand new watch.

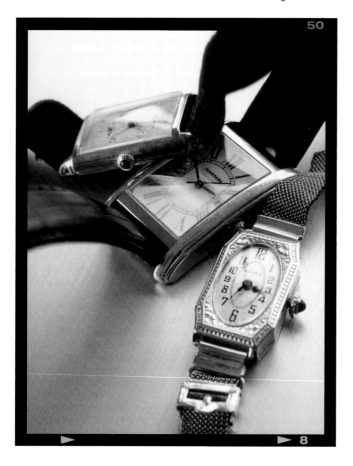

A cartoon-character watch face can make you snicker. Swatch watches are colorful, quirky, and inexpensive fun. On our first date, my husband wore a multicolored Swatch watch with his buttoned-up business suit. I loved the fact that he didn't need the Rolex gold.

A tailored man's watch gives a suggestion of power. Even the larger size watch bands can have a few additional holes punched in them, but worn a little loose they float on your arm and look interesting. My everyday watch is a man's tank.

A dainty jeweled evening watch dazzles. There are many beautiful antiques with filigreed silver or wonderful pink-gold from the past. Who cares if it keeps perfect time? There are many antique reproductions that look quite authentic.

Sports watches are pure, practical fun. The oversized dials, thick, colored, perforated rubber bands, and multidials have a strong look.

I replace the band on my antique gold watch with velvet or metallic ribbons to harmonize with whatever I am wearing. I tie it in a small bow and let the ends hang a bit. The touch of an unusual or interesting watch says volumes about the wearer.

SLEEVE PARTNERS

Bracelets are another way to add personality and color to your outfits. Whether you layer them over your watch or on one arm, just layer them. They are the perfect partners to pushed-up or rolled sleeves. Mixing and layering wide cuffs, chunky chains, geometrics, or sentimental charms make your individual style statement. Keep the styles, color tones, or themes consistent.

You can layer all platinum or all gold, or mix the gold, platinum, and a little bronze together. Metals no longer have to be one or the other. Cartier started the three-metal intertwined wedding band and broke the one-metal barrier. The more interesting the mix, the more interesting the wearer.

Charm bracelets are totally charming. You can collect your own individual charms over the years to tell the story of your life. Colorful plastics, wooden beads, flowers on fabric bands, any bracelets that you love make a good style statement.

THE LIGHTWEIGHTS

Earrings are one accessory that must change as we do. No matter how spectacular the earrings are, if they make your earlobes droop, they are doing you a major disservice. Whether clip or pierced, all your earrings should be lightweight. Clips need to fit on the ear, not stretch it down. Pierced earrings should never pull or tug. The only way to test earrings is to try them on. Some fabrications feel lightweight, until you wear them. Earrings are meant to add color and draw attention to your face.

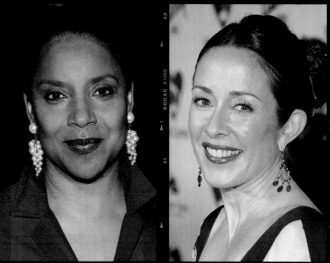

GROWN-UP GIRL'S EARRING RULE:

The longer the earring the more open the neckline. . . . I did not say lower!

Upturned collar, flattering color, and important, lightweight earrings are three positive face framers on Phylicia Rashad.

The heavyweights: Patricia Heaton in fabulous earrings, but how can you look past the drooping earlobes?

Don't match earrings to your necklaces; simply keep them in the same colors or metals. Have fun with earrings, change your styles, and play with color.

Display your earrings in a plastic compartmentalized hang-up bag in your closet. These come in all sizes depending on the size of your collection. You can easily find what you need quickly.

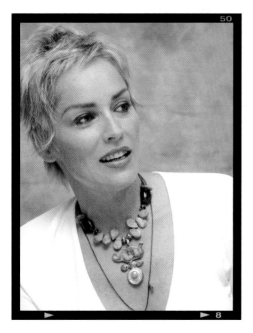

Multitasking jewelry at it's best on Sharon Stone. It's bold and defining and provides coverage.

Necklaces fall into two main categories: short and long. For in-between lengths, the only concern is the size of your bustline. A necklace that stops right at your bust will put emphasis on this area. If you are small-busted it can fill in, giving the appearance of a slightly larger bust. If you are full-busted it does the same.

If you wear long necklaces (anything more than 18 inches) you don't have to worry about your neck. Let your creativity and fun-loving spirit play with colors, textures, and mixes.

LINKS

Now that you're into long-sleeved shirts, buy a few with elegant French cuffs and borrow from men's style by adding cufflinks.

- French-braided fabric dots are inexpensive and come in all colors to match or complement your shirts.

- Pearl, diamond, or jeweled cufflinks are dressy.

- Whimsical cufflinks add mystery.

- Heirloom cufflinks add richness and tradition.

Plus or Minus Buttons

The secret to making buttons work for you is their placement on your body. Never put buttons where you don't want attention. Button pockets on our tushes or thighs? Why? Button pockets on our breasts? Only you know the answer to that one. Keep them strictly in the areas you want eyes to be looking. Vertical lines of buttons, down a blouse or jacket, are slimming. Horizontal buttons in decorative patterns can be widening.

Visit your local fabric store for buttons to upgrade your outfits. Please avoid the gimmicky buttons. Flower buttons look adorable on children, but on grown-up girls they look childish. Who wants to wear buttons that look like Dots gummy candy? I'd rather eat them.

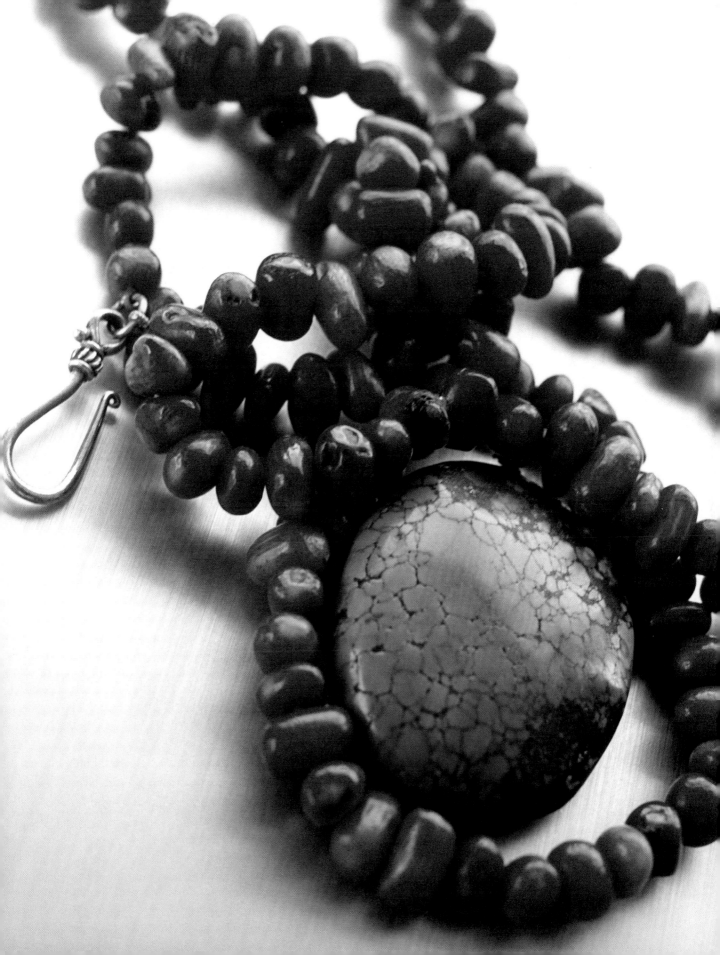

Specs

Love, love, love them! Just make sure they radiate style. The right glasses can make you look smart, the wrong ones can make you look dated. Take your best-dressed friend with you to select frames. Never depend on your own choice. Remember your eyes are either dilated or not corrected, so how can you tell what works? Most eyeglass experts are far from being experts in anything but fitting glasses. They are salespeople, not style people.

If you wear glasses on a daily basis, build a wardrobe. It's hard to find one pair of glasses that look right with everything. Watch for frame sales, visit antique shops, and garage sales to add to your glasses collection.

GROWN-UP GIRL'S GLASSES RULE:

Glasses are your #1 accessory priority.

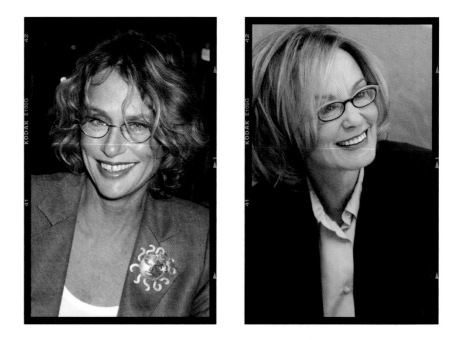

The word "practical" should only apply to your lens prescription. When it comes to choosing eyeglass frames, the word that comes to mind is "stylish." Nothing boring, utilitarian, or from five years ago. We want contemporary, fabulous looking glasses like those worn by Lauren Hutton and Jessica Lange.

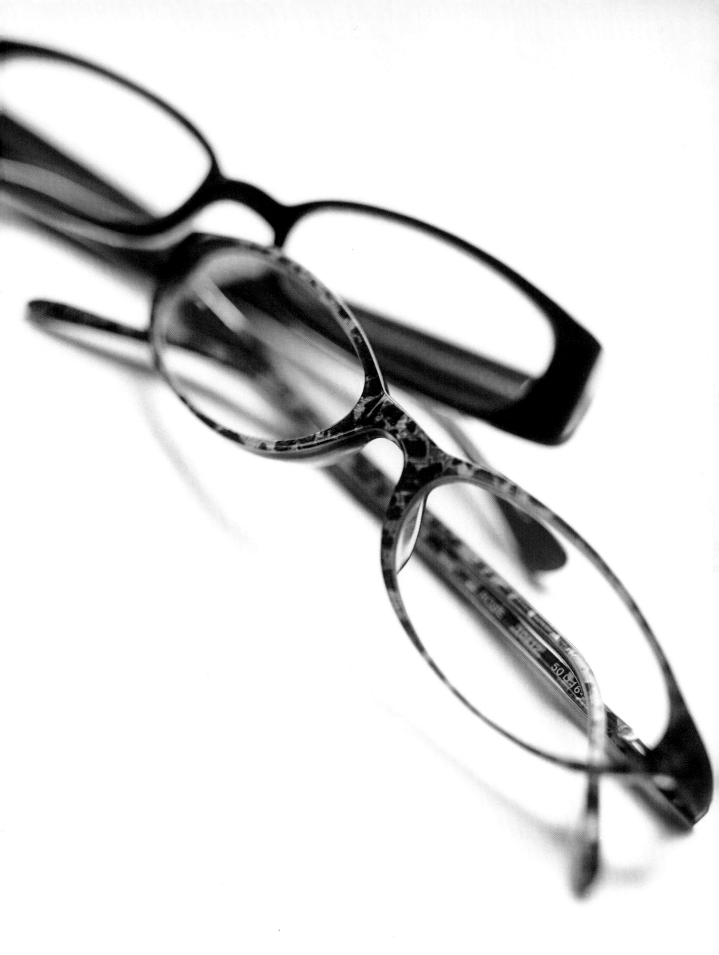

- **Classic frames:** A tortoise, black, or neutral-colored plastic that provides a professional attitude.

- **Blending frames:** A light-colored or clear plastic, rimless or thin metal frame that almost disappears on your face. Rimless can either work for you or make you appear older. Look closely at how the frame looks on you, not how much you like the look of the frame. Test them by standing back from a mirror. Move the glasses from your face to your hair—they should blend in with your hair color.

- **Funky frames:** Something unique that you absolutely adore. A bright red or purple plastic, or strong black horn-rims. They are unique in shape, size, and design. These frames will dominate your face and outfit, so wear them when your outfit is elegantly simple in both style and color. Of course, you should don them when you crave attention. All other accessories need to be nondescript.

- **Evening frames:** Delicate gold, silver, or bronze metal frames. Forgo ones with diamonds or jewels. Keep evening frames small and simple. Black tie does not mean dressed-up glasses.

Leave half glasses to college professors. They look distinguished peeking out over them; we just look old. If you only need correction for reading, opt for full blended bi-focals with clear glass in the upper half and your prescription in the lower half. You will look half the age of someone wearing half glasses. Avoid those tiny fold-up glasses that draw so many comments like "Where did you find those? They're amazing! And so practical." Do we ever want to look practical?

- **Never reveal that you are wearing bifocal or trifocal glasses** with that giveaway line between the different strengths. Spend the extra bucks and get the blended lenses; they are worth every single penny.

- **Today's frames are so fashionable that the shape of your face no longer determines their style.** The principle rule is to match your bone structure. If you are small-boned, go with smaller rims. If you are big-boned, balance your structure with larger frames.

- **Try glasses without the nose pads.** They don't leave those terrible indentations that can turn permanent.

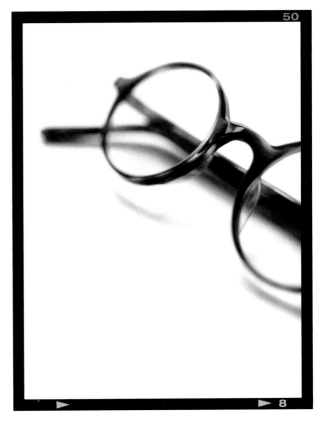

- **Remove any outdated glasses from your wardrobe.** Your choice of glasses reveals your attitude. Out-of-date glasses set the tone for your total appearance. Lenses with initials, gemstones, or decorative objects are from the seventies and should stay there.

- **Frame styles go in and out.** Aviator frames have made the rounds several times. We need to pass on them this round. Their egg shape once made us look cool, now it makes us look droopy. Oversized wraparounds are sleek and secretive when you're twenty. Now, they make us look like we just had our eyes dilated. Even Elton John has toned down his choices. So must we.

Today's selection of lenses is virtually unlimited. Follow these guidelines for the best looks:

- **Tinted lenses:** Stores love to sell you tinted lenses because they cost more. The only time you need tinted lenses is if you want a pair of glasses to run errands sans makeup. The most flattering tints are soft blues, warm ambers, and nudish pinks. The two G's, grays and greens, give a ghoulish tinge to skin tones.

- **Graduated tints:** Lenses that darken as the sun grows brighter, are one of our worst enemies. They never lighten to clear which means you have a gray or brown tint reflecting in your face at all times. You can't wear enough blush to balance this negative cast.

- **Contact lenses:** If you don't love frames, or need a break from glasses, this is your solution. With the new color contacts you can enhance or change your eye color. The caveat here is the intensity. Don't try to outblue Paul Newman. Only Elizabeth Taylor has lavender eyes. Softer and more natural is always better when it comes to eye color.

- **Mirrored lenses:** I prefer we keep our mirrors in our purses. Have you ever tried to have a real conversation with someone wearing mirrored lenses? It's like talking to yourself. I always end up checking my lipstick.

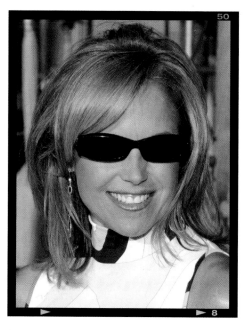

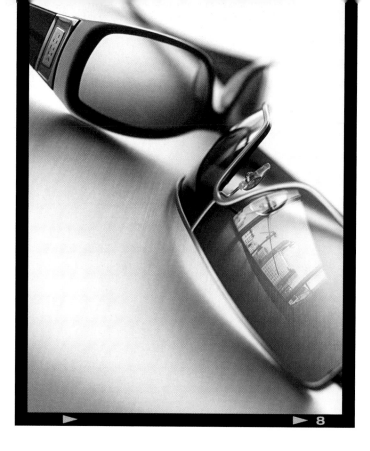

Who is that mysterious diva behind the sensuous shades? None other than television's own Katie Couric wearing a fabulous sunglass attitude.

• **Sunglasses:** Nothing adds more mystery, glamour, and drama than sunglasses. When choosing sunglasses, most of the basic eyeglass rules go out the window. Because the lenses are dark, you get to be more adventurous.

Sunglasses allow you to observe without being observed. Pick your frames according to your purpose. Do you want the celebrity factor? Nothing does it better than black. Do you want standout shades? Try juicy orange frames or high-wattage red.

Avoid the high-tech cyberchic sunglasses. We are not interested in being one of the Bond girls. Don't wear your initials or your birth sign etched on your lenses—you know who you are. Beware of too many studded crystals on the frames. A little crystal adds a little sparkle and that's all we need, just a little.

GROWN-UP GIRL'S SUNGLASSES RULE:

Sunglasses must look like they belong on your face. Don't select frames by what is the "latest," go with frames that make you look the "greatest."

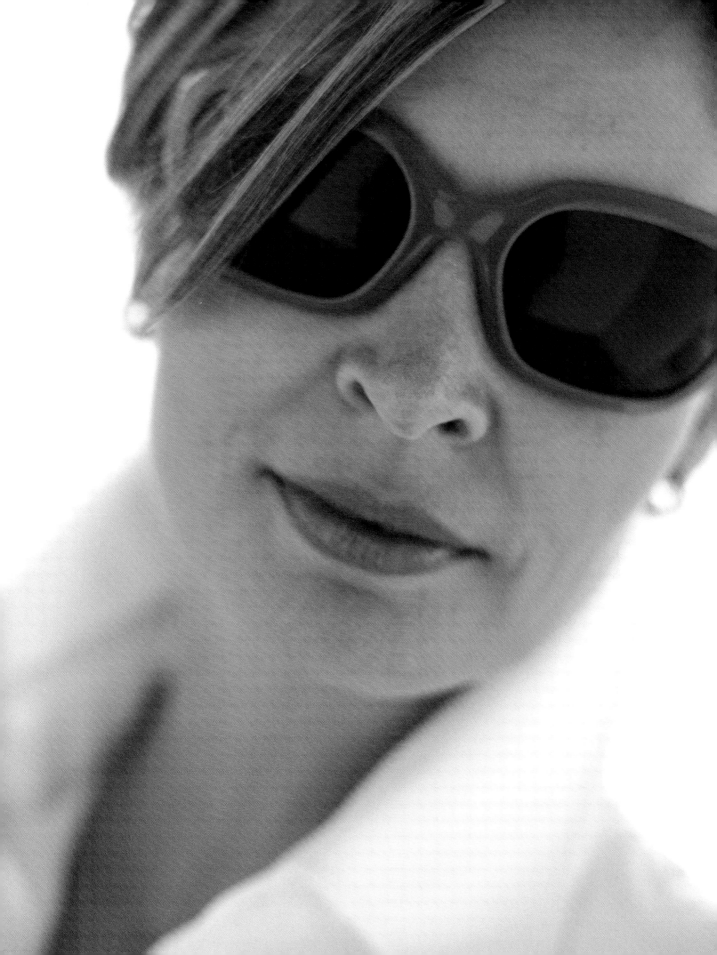

Under the Queen's Hat

First ask yourself if you are a hat person. You will know the answer by the number of hats in your closet, and not the ones gathering dust. If you are, then you already know the advantages of plopping on a baseball, bucket, or raffia hat when you're having a bad hair day. Hats create a look. They protect you from the sun while they frame and flatter your face. Casual hats are cool. Dressy hats require the proper event to warrant them.

Hats are fun, practical, and affordable. Soft, foldable hats are perfect for travel. They pack easily and fit into your coat pocket or bag for touring. You can handle any weather condition—heat, wind, or rain—with your hat. I like the ones with the 2 to 3-inch brims. The brim can protect you from sun and hide your hair from humidity or rain damage. Turn the back brim up and leave the front brim down to shield your eyes. Turn the front brim up and leave the back brim down for focus on your face. Buy solid colors. Just like shirts, prints are too busy by your face.

GROWN-UP GIRL'S HAT RULE:

"When you wear a hat, don't wear a hairstyle." Your hair needs to be pulled back, up, or brushed softly down.

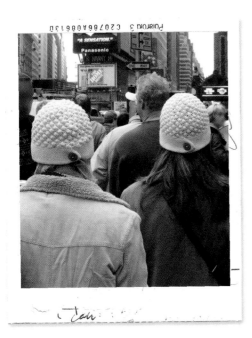

It's great to shop with a friend, but stop there. Who wants to look like a matched pair?

Avoid the matronly hat and glove look. If the hat looks like it is balancing on the top of your hair or you are attending the Kentucky Derby, get rid of it. Queen Elizabeth is not our role model.

Hillary's Big Don't

All I need to say here is "Hillary Clinton's headbands." Leave the hair accessories to the teenagers. Wear a simple clip or coated rubber band if you must, but otherwise, please don't decorate your hair. Decorate your house, your garden, and your cakes— these all benefit from a little enhancement. Our hair needs to stand alone, unadorned.

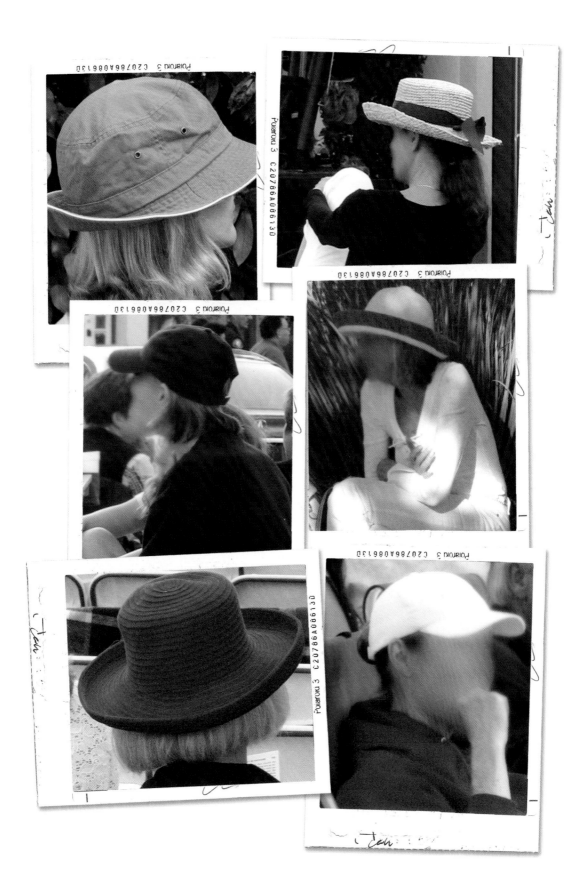

Gender Benders

Ties are my favorite gender-bender accessories. Nothing punches up a shirt like a great stripe, polka dot, or floral tie. For our purposes ties only work with tailored clothing: a power suit, a shirtwaist dress, or a genteel skirt and blouse. If you are petite, buy your ties in the boy's department. The scale is slightly smaller and so is the price. Avoid ties if you are bosomy. Extra padding is not the accessory you need.

GROWN-UP GIRL'S ACCESSORY RULE:
Don't try for too many accessory style statements at once.

Less is always best. Accessories are the icing on the cake. They are meant to complete your outfit, and help cover up areas that need covering in a fashionable way. As our wardrobe choices pare down, our accessories become our personal style statements. Look at your accessories—what statement are they making about you?

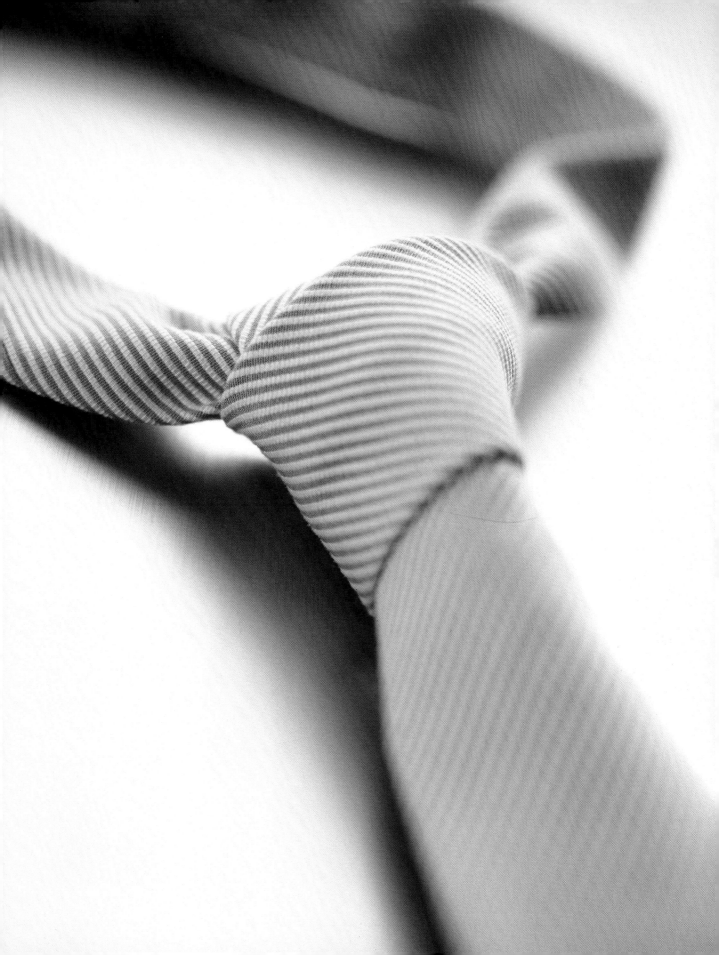

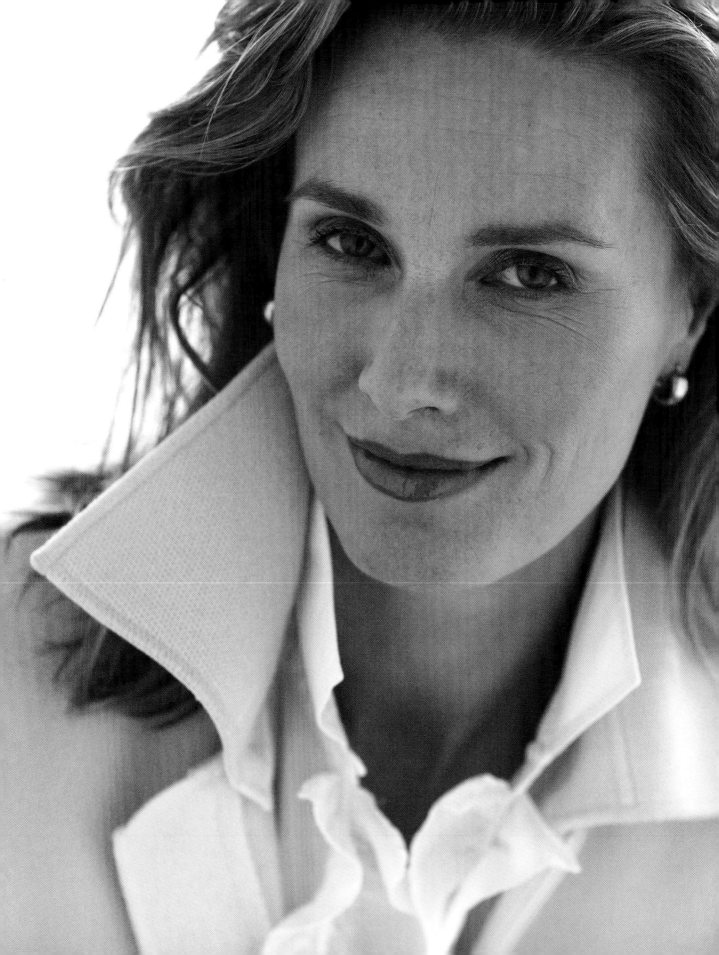

PART TWO

Beauty

Beauty is the most desired word associated with women. Who doesn't want to be considered beautiful? What makes a woman beautiful? To listen to advertisers you would think it's a treatment cream, a makeup product, or a medical procedure. Indeed, in today's world, it can be. Beauty is inherited, but it's also acquired and perfected with technology. Can any woman be beautiful? I think she can come very close. We live in a time of incredible products and amazing procedures. We don't have to age like our predecessors, we can age as gracefully as we desire. It's a new era in beauty and we are the lucky recipients.

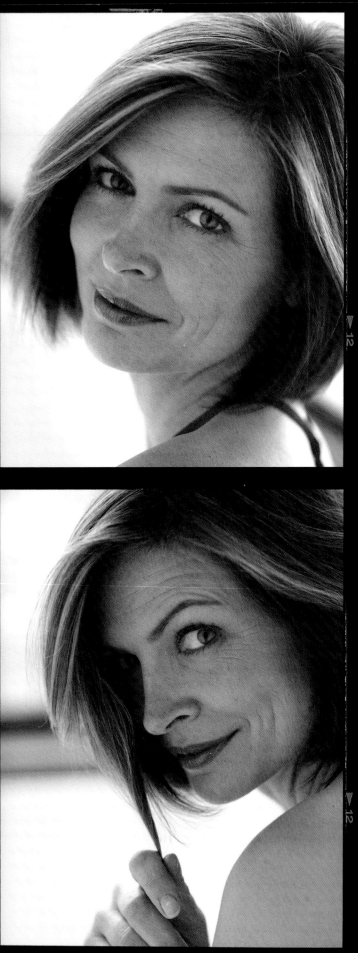
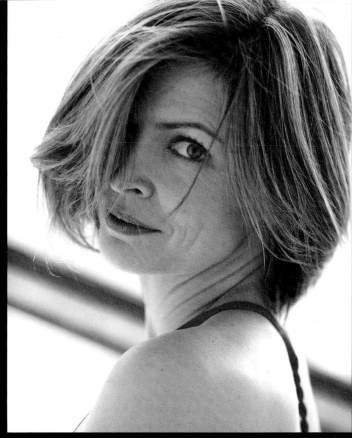
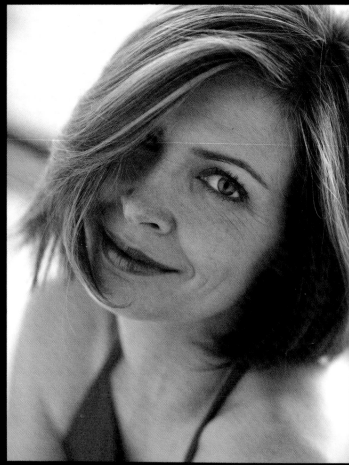

CHAPTER FIVE

Hair

I admit I have a hair obsession, and I am confident in saying that I am not alone. Most of the women I know suffer from the same obsession. We see our hair as a universal, ageless problem. We spend money, time, and energy trying to achieve "perfect hair days." I don't know anyone, well, hardly anyone, who doesn't feel better about themselves when they are having a good hair day. It is an ongoing search for the right hairdresser, the best style, and the appropriate products to maintain that style.

My philosophy is to deal with the hair you have, not the hair you want to have. I spent years yearning for thick, wavy hair. I finally got real. I have thin hair with two cowlicks in my bangs and three at my crown. Humid weather gives my hair its own creative look that only a hat can save. Talk about a challenge!

When I finally learned to accept what I have and make the best of it, I was able to control my hair most of the time. Controlling your hair all the time means you are doing something unfashionably wrong. We want our hair to look soft and pretty, not molded and sprayed. The older we get the more soft and natural our hair should be. I don't believe you can have good hair without maintenance. Wash-and-wear styles look like wash-and-wear styles to me. "All I do is get up in the morning and run my fingers through my hair" looks like that's all you did.

We are all slaves to our hair. My goal is to free us from bondage. We don't have the same hair in texture or style we had at twenty. We don't want it to look exactly like it did when we were thirty. We need it to look good now: appropriate, stylish, and contemporary.

Poodles and Helmets

I love poodles. I just don't love the poodle cut, or any short, boring, practical cut to which women tend to gravitate as they mature. Sure, it's easy to maintain. Whenever I go to a movie theater, I look at the back of women's heads. I can almost always guess their ages by their hair. The older the woman, the shorter the hair. When I see "sleep" indentations on the back of those heads I want to scream. Don't they realize we are multidimensional?

I am all for helmets for protection in sports. I am totally against them in hairstyles. Does your hair move with the wind, and I don't mean in all one piece like Donald Trump's? Can you run your fingers through it? Is it soft and shiny? Is your hairstyle contemporary? If you answer no to any of these questions, it's time for a change.

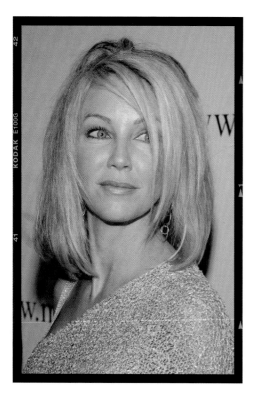

Heather breaks the myth. Her shoulder-length hair is gorgeous, gorgeous, gorgeous.

GROWN-UP GIRL'S HAIR RULE:

Don't believe that older age has to mean shorter hair. I am at this very moment breaking the beauty myth that forty is the cutoff time for longer hair. Forty is the time for good hair, whatever length.

Five or six years ago, I was bored with my various versions of the "bob." It was time to do something drastic. Always liking the tousled hair of Meg Ryan, I decided that was the new look for me. I found the best hair designer for that cut and made my appointment. It took forever because he is a celebrity in his own right, but I waited. By the time my appointment came I was so ready. Cut, blown-dry, moussed-out, tousled, there it was . . . Meg Ryan hair. I loved it. I left feeling on top of the world.

When meeting a group of friends for dinner that night they all commented on my new do. "Wow, you really made a big change." "Is it hard to get your hair to stick out like that?" "You look so much . . . hipper." Thank you, thank you, thank you. I was so in love with the cut that I really thought these were compliments.

The next morning my hair looked like a flattened bubble. Not to worry, I added my new product called "Dirt" and it stuck out all over once again. (I should have known that any hairstyle that requires a product called Dirt is probably not the one I want.) It took me about a week to realize I had made a big mistake.

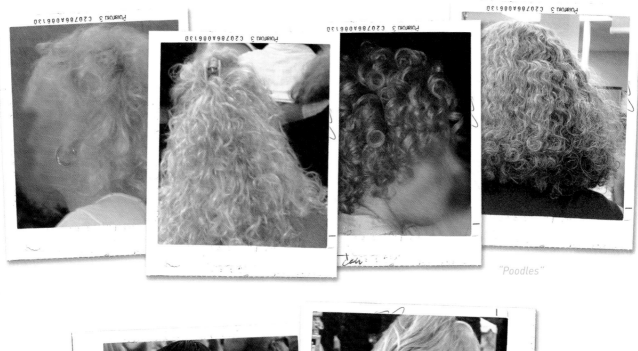

"Poodles"

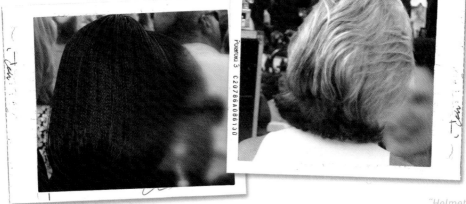

"Helmets"

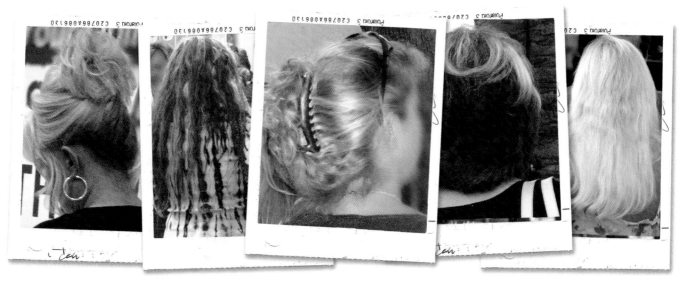

"Time Capsules"

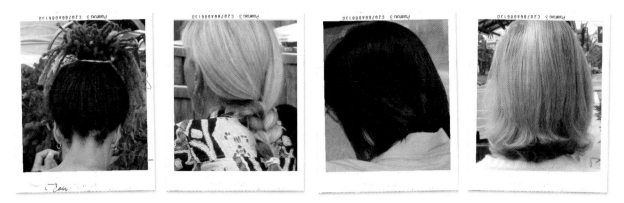

You may not be able to tell our grown-up girls' exact ages from the back of these heads, but you can tell they are contemporary and chic.

It was a great haircut, contemporary haircut, great hair designer, just not the right look for me. Once I got over the excitement of the change I realized that I am not Meg Ryan. Neither my hair texture nor my lifestyle is like Meg Ryan's. It took me about a year to grow out all the layers. Last week as I sat in my hair designer's chair checking out the back of the newest version of my bob, there sat Meg Ryan in the next chair, waiting her turn. I still love her messed-up hair . . . but now, I love it *on her*.

HAIR FASHION MYTH: "LONG HAIR IS AGING. IT DRAGS YOU DOWN. SHORT HAIR IS UPLIFTING."

Jackie Kennedy got it right—she never cut her hair into a poodle cut. She knew the value of a little length. Length equals softness. Length enables you to have some sort of style. I'm not talking long straight hair. Length can mean a longer bang, a one-length short bob, or a little turned-up fringe in the back. I'm talking soft, styled, contemporary hair.

There are options for short hair other than a poodle cut. Ellen DeGeneres wears short hair on the longer side. It softens and complements her chic tailored style. Diane Sawyer wears stylish shorter hair, but it's the opposite of the poodle and the helmet. Katie Couric has grown out her once-practical short hair to a shoulder-length do that moves and glistens under the TV cameras.

Most of us need softness. Most of us need style. Most of us need a little more hair. Forget all those pictures that show face shapes and recommended hairstyles. They make great magazine copy and fill a lot of pages in beauty books. With each decade we require a little more softness, regardless of the shape of our face. Oblong, square, round, who really cares? If you have contemporary hair it will blow and move with the breeze, revealing your true face shape. What matters is the end result.

GROWN-UP GIRL'S HAIRSTYLE RULE:

Trendier hair does not translate to younger-looking hair.

Trendier hair might make you look sillier. What you want is a blending of the classic and current styles. Bridget Bardot and Ann Margret big hair are making a comeback. Just as in fashion, if you were around for the real deal you should probably skip the rerun. The only thing worse than the back-of-the-head poodle cuts in the movie theater is the youthful cutting-edge cut that turns around and reveals a face that doesn't match. The balance lies somewhere in between.

Your Perfect Mate

If you're thinking you already found your perfect mate, great, but unless he or she is able to give you the best haircut you have ever had, keep looking. There is room in your life for two perfect mates, and one of them must own scissors, probably sport tattoos, and perhaps have "distinctive" hair.

No woman's life is totally complete without a fabulous hair designer, and I am talking the best. Having owned and operated a trendsetting salon for seven years, I know the reason the top stylists charge more is because they are worth it. Their talent is in demand. You have to plan your life around their availability and then take a second loan on your house to pay them. A good haircut can make your daily hairstyling life easier. It can make you look contemporary, and it simply looks and feels good.

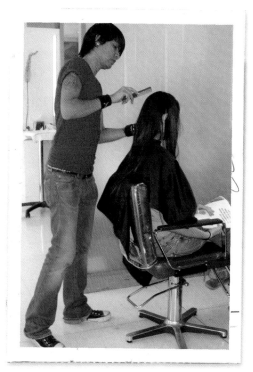

You know the minute you see Cervando that he will keep your hair moving forward.

How do you find the stylist of your dreams?

- *You ask women.* If you see a great-looking haircut on someone, stop and ask who did it. Flattery will get you sources.
- *Try different designers.* Hair grows back. Don't use the same person for years on end. They will end up letting you influence them and that usually leads to time-warp hair.
- *Read about good salons and stylists.* Newspapers or fashion and beauty magazines do the research for you.

- *Look at the designer.* You are in trouble if she looks like your mother or dresses like your aunt.
- *Visit local salons.* You can tell by the location, decor, clientele, and the cars in the parking lot if it is a top salon. You may drive a Honda, but you want a Lexus on your head.

Once you have found your perfect mate:

- Make them look at you in your clothes, as opposed to the tentlike capes they use to cover you.
- Tell them what you like and dislike about your hair.
- Bring pictures of magazine models whose look you like in all aspects, not just hair. This gives them an idea of how you perceive yourself.
- Listen and be open to their suggestions. They want to please you because this translates into tips and they live for tips.
- Don't chat. The client in the chair on your left may be getting her psychotherapy while the client on your right is reviewing movies. Keep quiet and let them concentrate on your hair.
- If you love your hair, tip, tip, and tip. They always remember who tips and it's amazing how that translates into "emergency" appointment accommodations.
- Give them a call. Not to make an appointment, just to leave a message saying you love your hair. Everyone likes compliments.
- If you are not satisfied after doing everything right, go back in and have a conversation prefaced with "You are a terrific hair designer and I'm not criticizing you. It is probably my lack of skills, but I am having a hard time working with this hairstyle." Okay, so you don't mean it and you want to rant and rave. I promise you this conversation will make them help you, not hate you. You don't want someone who is angry working on your head with scissors. If that fails, speak with the manager and ask for your money back, then start the search process all over.

Working in the Neil George Salon in Beverly Hills is celebrity hair designer Cervando Maldonado. As a stylist for Goldie Hawn, Rosanna Arquette, Gina Gershon, and John Bon Jovi, Cervando is always on some type of fashion shoot. His clientele is a combination of the celebrity and the noncelebrity. Here are some of Cervando's thoughts on hair for the grown-up girl:

- If longer hair looks good on you, keep it, but keep it appropriate. If longer hair makes you feel youthful and sexy, make it work for you at the age you are now.
- Have a little volume at the roots, even with straight hair. This is softer and more flattering than completely flat hair.
- Modify the trends so they are natural and complementary, rather than over the top. Too trendy looks out of place. Have confidence in the way you look.
- Hair should always be age appropriate. Keep it sophisticated and au courant without copying your daughter's hairstyle.
- Make sure all your elements match: hair, face, clothes, and lifestyle.
- Find a hairdresser who wants to work with you, will listen to you, and bring your look into modern times.

Cervando's Products

Here is What You Will Find on Cervando's Styling Station:

For shine:

- L'Oreal Relaxed by Kerastase for thicker hair. Leaves incredible shine and softness.
- Dr. Hauschka's Neem Oil for a deep conditioning treatment. Even left on the hair for seconds before washing, you will get benefits.
- Rene Furterer Leave-In Conditioner—adds a little volume as well.

For thickening:

- Phyto Volume gives life and still leaves your hair soft.
- Big Sexy Hair is a great root-lifter for fine, limp hair.
- Sebastian Mousse Fizz XL for that spiky Meg Ryan hair.

About tools:

- Always buy the best tools you can.

Blow dryers:

- Super Solano—most hairdressers' favorite, including mine. The best dryer when you want stick-straight hair.
- Chi Ionic dryer, dries fastest while protecting the hair.

Irons:

- Hot Tools Curling Iron—has a temperature gauge to prevent burning.
- Beeza Flat Iron—gets hot enough to only need one time per spot. Velvet covering lets you get close to scalp and face.

GROWN-UP GIRL'S HAIR PRODUCT RULE:

Rotate products for maximum results. When a product stops working, start shopping.

A little hair product goes a long way. One of the most common mistakes in home hairstyling is the overuse of treatment and styling aides. Too many products or too much of one product can weigh your hair down. To get the perfect results for your hair texture and style, introduce products one at a time. Start with the smallest amount possible. If the first product works but you need a bit more of something else, add the second item the next time you shampoo. It's easier to work your way into products rather than having to rewash your hair because it's overloaded with "stuff."

Tool Time

When it comes to hair tools there are not a lot of major changes between what you used at twenty and what you use now. It all depends on your hairstyle. The only important factor is that hair ages and it ages more rapidly when it is overheated. Every tool we use makes some type of heat and this is where we do the damage.

In a hurry in the morning? Your blow dryer on hot dries a lot faster than medium, but it also does a lot more damage.

Hair too curly? Flat irons straighten it out while they cook your ends if you don't have one with heat controls.

Need some curls? Curling irons do the trick and fry your ends as well if you don't feed the hair in from the middle of the shaft. Hot rollers focus the heat on the ends of your hair unless you first wrap those ends in end papers.

Ends, Ends, Ends! It's the ends that get the majority of the damage because they get the majority of the heat. Hopefully, you cut off the ends on a regular basis, but if you

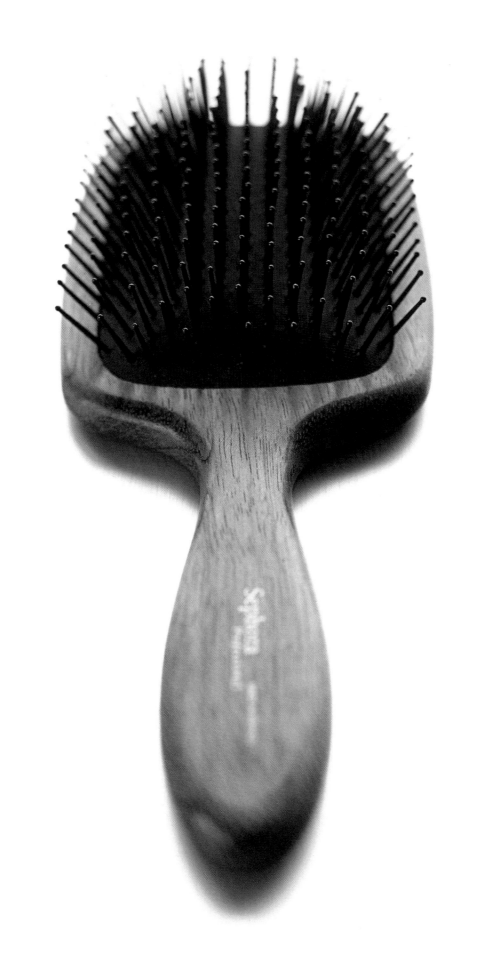

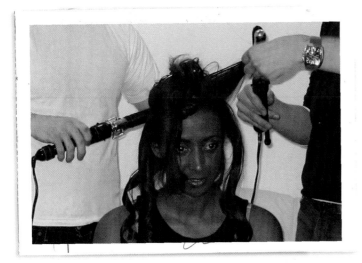

Is this not every woman's dream of the perfect threesome?

cut off all the damage you will end up with one of those dreadful poodle or helmet hair-dos. Forget about it. You can cut them off, treat them with conditioners to make the appearance look slightly better, or prevent the damage in the first place. It's all about prevention.

HAIR FASHION MYTH: "YOU CAN REPAIR SPLIT ENDS."

The biggest improvements in hair tools are the ionic blow dryers, flat irons, and brushes. The ionic head has more sheen, less damage, and less fizzy frizz. Fizzy is only good in our cocktails of choice.

GROWN-UP GIRL'S HAIRSTYLING TOOL RULE:
Update your styling implements. The new technology can save you time as well as save your hair.

The Greyhound Bus

Get off the bus immediately. Forget that you have earned every gray hair on your head. My goal is to keep you looking on the outside the way you feel on the inside. I can't do that with gray hair. I know many women who have beautiful gray hair. It's thick, shiny, and show-stopping. Only it's gray and gray just adds on ten years. I don't care how young your face looks or how great you dress, gray says "older" which is not a bad thing, but it is a strong statement.

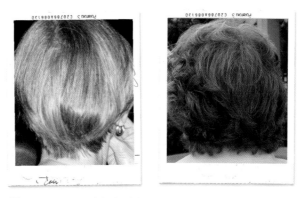

These grown-up girls don't have to turn around, you already know their ages.

If you are gray because you love it, terrific. If you are gray because you have given up, I say color, color, color. If you do have that fabulous gray hair, it will still be there at a later date if you desire to be natural into your sunset years.

The secret to coloring hair is to make it look natural. Sharon Osborne looks incredible with her fuchsia streaks. Cher looks thirty regardless of what color her hair is. (Of course, we would all look thirty if we followed her costly regimen of maintenance.)

Hair Color Basics

Stick to these basic hair color principles:

- Natural means several colors blended together, not one solid mass. Look at the coloring on children's heads.
- Natural means shine. Nature, years, heat, and chemicals take away shine. The good news is you can now buy temporary shine in a bottle, jar, or spray container.
- As you get older, go *slightly* lighter if you have dark hair. Just don't go to that bleached blonde that resembles white. If you have light hair add a little depth for a richer look.
- Keep colors in the warm and natural tones: golden hues, honey tints, warm toffees. Stay away from icy blondes, ash browns, charcoal blacks, and artificial reds.
- If you think that little bit of gray is looking like blonde highlights, look again. It probably just looks gray. Gray sprinkles throughout your hair tend to dull even the shiniest hair underneath.
- Find the best colorist by using the same methods listed under finding the best hair designer.

BEAUTY FASHION MYTH: "GRAY HAIR IS BEAUTIFUL."

On men and dogs it may indeed be beautiful, but on you, it is aging. Are you ready for that?

GROWN-UP GIRL'S HAIR COLOR RULE:

Once you commit to hair color, commit. Maintenance is the key. Stretching your root touch-up an additional week means wearing a hat to cover the evidence. Roots are never attractive. Keep all the roots in your garden.

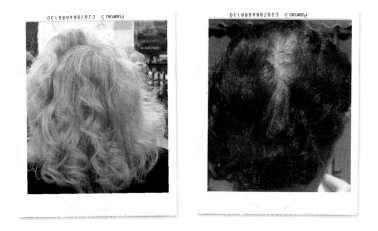

Just a bit too long between color and everyone knows you're not the natural grown-up girl they thought you were.

The Color Neophyte

The majority of hair color is done at home. It has been made affordable, easy-to-use, and multitasking because you can cook or clean while it processes—just don't answer the door. The pictures of the luxurious hair models on the boxes make anyone want to copy them. The names of the colors are so delicious: who wouldn't want to be known as the "Caribbean Carmel" brunette, or a "Ginger Twist" redhead?

The important question here is how do you get natural-looking color at home? If you can't visit the best, I am bringing the best to you. Lorri Goddard-Clark is one of the leading hair colorists in the country. Working out of the Neil George Salon in Beverly Hills, her clientele includes: Drew Barrymore, Kim Basinger, the Olsen twins (Mary-Kate and Ashley), Kate Capshaw, and Denise Richards.

Lorri can take you out of the home haircolor box and turn your hair color into professional-looking color. Here are some of her tips:

- Keep it simple. Don't get into major procedures, major highlights, or corrective color. This is where you need a professional.
- Stay within a few shades of your natural hair color.
- To cover gray, you don't have to go lighter; too light or too bright will wash you out.
- Don't get trendy with color. Stay with chic, sexy, believable colors.
- For the first attempt, if in doubt, do a test strand. Cut a small piece—about twenty hairs—from the back of your head and color. Use your math to reduce

the amount of color, just like adjusting down a recipe. This will enable you to see what you are getting without coloring your entire head.

- Write down your formulas and keep them inside the color boxes.

- Always buy two boxes of color.

    - *The first one is your recipe color and should be a shade lighter than the color for which you are aiming. Always select lighter colors, it's easier to go darker than to lighten dark hair.*

    - *The second is your "spice" color. Blondes, try a warm light brown. Brunettes should use a rich nutmeg color. Redheads might add a golden brown. Black hair needs a rich, deep brown spice.*

- You will have to play with the formulas. Try 7/8 parts recipe color to 1/8 part spice color. Adjust as you go along. Your hair color recipe is like a cooking recipe. You have to tweak it to your own perfection.

- If you have resistant gray, add 2 to 3 drops of Ardell Gray Magic to your formula. (available at www.Aiibeauty.com)

- Highlighting kits: You must focus on the regrowth only. Don't keep pulling through to the ends (this includes blondes and brunettes). You will end up with ends that are overbleached and damaged. The only exception is redheads, they should always pull through to the ends. A few pieces around the face are more believable than a head of highlights. Don't overdo it.

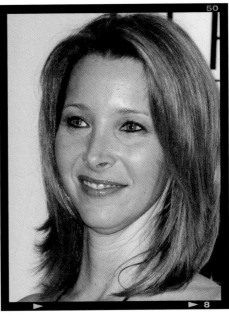

- Things to avoid with home color:

    - *Pink shades of red.*

    - *Overhighlighted blondes.*

    - *Harsh black. Even if your hair color is black, a shade lighter will be softer as you age.*

    - *If you get a color you can't live with:*

        Mix 1/2 cup Prell shampoo with 1 tablespoon baking soda. Shampoo hair. Rinse really, really well. Deep condition with a strong reconditioner like John Frieda's Kelp Hair or Wella's Cholesterol. Repeat the shampoo once a day until you remove enough of the color to recolor.

Lisa Kudrow exchanged very blond hair for natural-looking blonde hair. Is she growing up?

- For emergency touch ups: mix just enough to color your hairline and part. One quarter of your normal formula should do the trick. If there is any left, use it on your brows.

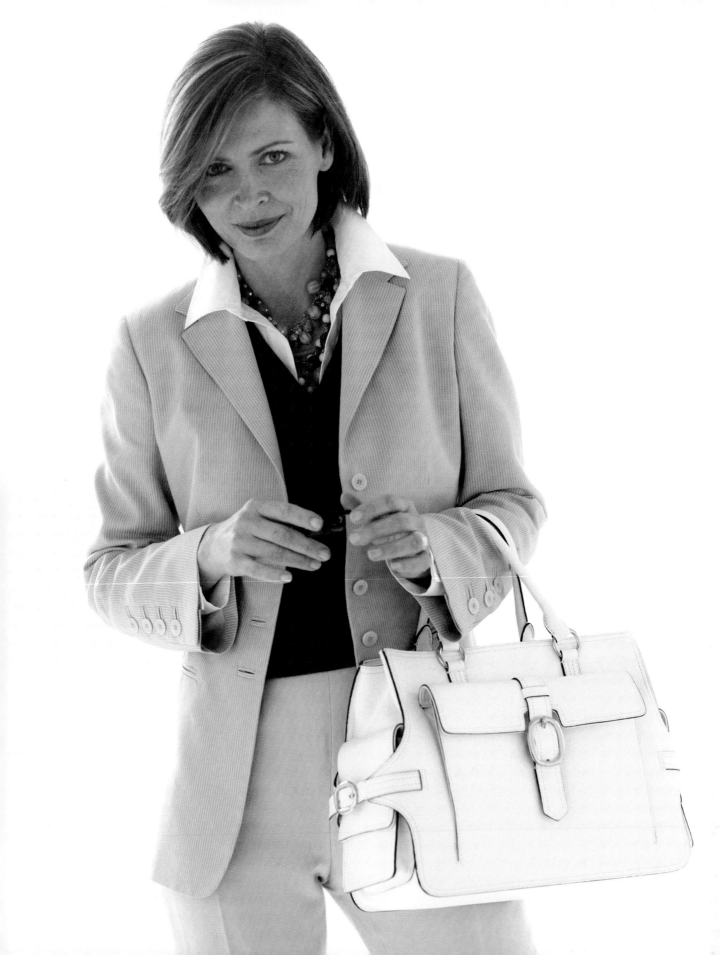

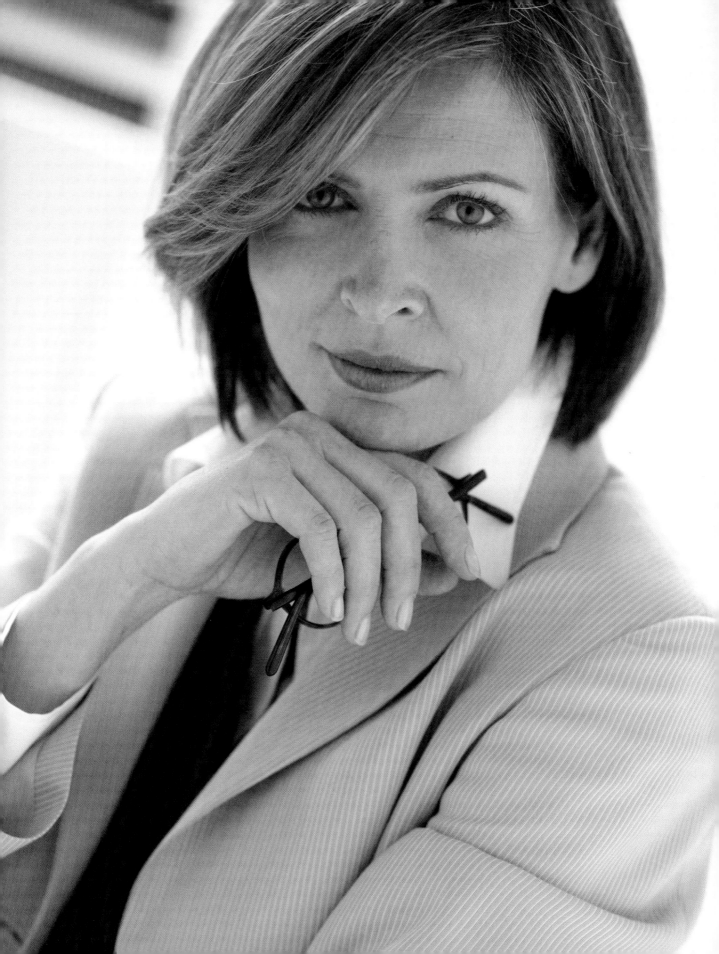

- L'Oreal, Clairol, Wella—it's all about what is easily available in the stores in your neighborhood.
- ARTec Color Shampoos for maintaining and enriching color.
- Goldwell Color Mousse instead of rinses. Most rinses take away the luster of the hair as they add color.
- Maybelline eye pencils work for in between touch-ups. Rub a soft toothbrush over the color and then apply to your regrowth. If you can't get a pencil in your color, try flat powder eye shadows. Both give the illusion of coverage. If you keep your hands away from the area, this should last until you shampoo.

Fat Hair

Oh how I yearn for fat hair, those thick, luxurious ringlets of Nicole Kidman, Amy Irving, or Mary Steenburgen. I even love the way they look pulled up and back in a simple ponytail holder, with curly wisps framing their faces. That's because my ponytail is too

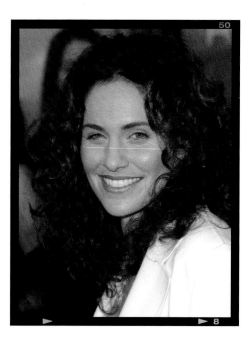

Do you think Amy Brenneman appreciates her fat hair as much as I do?

thin for anything other than a children's-size holder. I followed Dyan Cannon around a health food market one day just to look at her beautiful blonde curls close up. She thought I was looking at the organic strawberries. Yet I have friends who spend thousands of dollars trying to tame their manes, which they describe as unruly, wild, and frizzy. They complain of aching backs and arms from trying to blow-dry their hair. They would gladly trade with me. If only . . .

Fat hair can be controlled with product, blow-dryers, and flat irons. It just takes patience, practice, and trial testing of products. What works for one is not what works for all.

When it comes to chemical straightening such as the much-talked-about Japanese Straightening Treatment, the jury is still out. Some women feel it changed their life, some feel it ruined their hair. What's the difference? First, the technician: you must go to someone who does *only* straightening. You want a specialist, not a hairstylist who just took a weekend seminar. Second, you must understand that chemicals of any kind are inconsistent. The first process will probably be wonderful, because your hair is virgin. The second process can dull and damage a little, but it's still worth the straightness. The question comes into play with the additional treatments. How much damage are you willing to have in lieu of curls? Remember that forty-plus hair is not the same as twenty-something hair. If you color your hair you add another factor. You can only do one-process base color. Any highlights are very risky. The best colorist will tell you to proceed with extreme caution and only do a few small areas around the face. They may name the chemical process with positive sounding names like "thermal reconditioners," but they are chemicals and like color and perms, they do damage with repeat performances.

Skinny Hair

Is aging nature's hair diet? I was blow-drying my hair one morning, when I realized I could see right through my bangs to my round brush. Where were my bangs? It happened so gradually that I didn't realize it at first. I immediately made an appointment with my dermatologist, who, after testing me, said quite simply "Your hair is thinning. Is there any baldness in your family?" Yikes, my father was bald and my mother's hair is so thin she wears wigs.

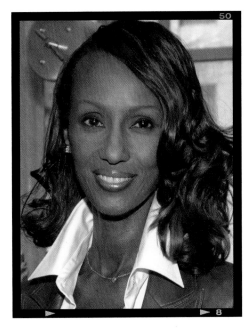

Iman combines great color with straightening and the look is beautifully natural.

How could I be a bald television fashion reporter? I would have to hire my own makeup artist just to keep my head powdered! I might have to avail myself of the camouflage products the television studio's hairstylist uses. (It appears to be hairspray but is actually colored spray to cover balding scalps—think spray paint!) Many powders and lotions thicken hair while covering the scalp or actually add little fibers to your hair, like lash-building mascara. I thought those items were only for men! Using my investigative skills I found out that nearly 80 percent of women have significant thinning in the front of their head.

While looking for the best expert for an *Entertainment Tonight* interview, Dr. Walter Unger was the name I heard over and over. He is a clinical professor at Mt. Sinai Medical School in New York City, a visiting professor at Johns Hopkins Medical School in Baltimore, and an associate professor at the University of Toronto. He is considered the guru of hair loss.

If your hair is on the skinny diet, here's what Dr. Walter Unger recommends:

- First, see a dermatologist who specializes in hair problems. He or she will examine you and do blood work to find out if a medical disorder is the cause of your hair loss.

- Second, try cosmetic camouflage treatments:

– Hair Magic—Keratin protein fibers

– DermMatch—Topical shading powder

– COUVRe—Alopecia masking lotion

– ProTHIK—aerosol hair thickening system

- Third, look at your diet. Carbs, fats, and crash diets rob you of protein. Add essential protein by eating meat, fowl, fish, cheese, and milk.

- Fourth, talk to your doctor about medical treatments, for example, using Propecia and 5 percent Minoxidil together. Propecia is safe for women as long as you are not pregnant or don't become pregnant. Use this combination for a year and see if you get results. Have your blood tested throughout the year.

- Fifth, investigate surgical hair transplants.

Here are Dr. Unger's tips on hair loss and transplanting:

- Frequent washing of your hair does not cause hair loss. If anything it does the opposite. Keep your head free of grease, dirt, and oil.

- If you have any question whether you are getting enough vitamins and minerals, get a good one-a-day vitamin and mineral supplement.

- Find a physician whose primary interest is the causes and treatments of hair loss. In general, family doctors and some dermatologists don't know that much about hair restoration surgery. Hair transplanting surgery for women is so much better than it used to be, even five to ten years ago, and many doctors are not aware of the advances.

- Don't spend tons of money on junk products; locate a good doctor. Don't look around for miracles. Products advertised in magazines and newspapers have probably not undergone double-blind, controlled, independent scientific studies. If a product works, they won't have to advertise. Word of mouth will have people banging down their doors.

- After you have tried cosmetic treatments and medical treatments, search for a specialist in hair transplanting.

- You know you have the right doctor if he/she is realistic about expectations. It takes between one and three sessions to restore hair to a reasonable density. You know you have the wrong doctor if he or she tries to accomplish too much too quickly. Any doctor that recommends overly "dense packing" or very large "megasessions" of grafts is not the doctor for you. You may want to do it as quickly as possible, but this is not where you want to save time.

You can get the same results in two conventional sessions as in one session of "dense packing," but without the damage to existing hair that may occur with the latter.

- If the transplanting is done right, you will see a noticeable increase in hair density in the area treated and no existing hair will have been removed.

GROWN-UP GIRL'S FACIAL HAIR RULE:

Get rid of it.

Wanton Hair

We can't resist running our hands over those adorable, downy baby heads. However when that same hair turns up on our upper lips, cheeks, and chins there is nothing irresistible about it. It's not cute on our faces, it's aging. We need to get rid of it, quickly.

There are many products and treatments on the market to remove or lighten facial hair. I don't recommend lightening although the facial bleaches do work, if you want light hair on your face instead of dark hair. It won't show in the comfort of a softly lit room. The problem is, we are not in softly lit rooms all the time. We are seen in bright sunlight, fluorescent light, and harsh overhead light. So skip right over the bleaching products and go for the removal ones.

I have tried the European threading method (a technician uses a taut thread to pull out facial hair) that Cher is a fan of and it works, but it's only as good as your technician. Even the best technicians miss areas and there you are, checking your makeup in your rearview mirror and finding a missed patch on your left cheek.

The best methods for facial hair removal are waxing, depilatories, electrolysis, and lasers. It is important to find out all you can about your options before choosing one that is right for you.

WAXING

Do-it-yourself home waxing or professional salon waxing both do the same thing. It's important to use the gentle wax designed especially for the face.

- Test facial wax first. Many skins are too sensitive and you may end up removing a thin layer of skin along with the hair, especially on the delicate upper lip.
- If you do it yourself, wash your hands first and keep your hands off your face after you're finished.
- Don't immediately apply makeup over the waxed areas.

DEPILATORIES

There are depilatories made especially for the face. They are far gentler than those designed for the body.

- Test first because they can be irritating.
- Protect your lips from burning with a lip treatment product like ChapStick before you apply the depilatory cream.
- Watch your time; if four to seven minutes is recommended, start with four. You can burn the skin if you leave it on too long.
- If you don't leave it on long enough, repeat the next day. *Never* use a depilatory twice in one day.
- Never use on irritated or broken-out skin.
- Follow the directions on the box. These are not experimental products.

ELECTROLYSIS

Anything with an electronic needle needs serious consideration. If waxing and depilatories don't fill your needs, this is the next and hopefully final step. It's all about the technician. You must do your homework and find the most qualified professional. Done properly, electrolysis removes hair at the root permanently. Done incorrectly, it scars the face. Your doctor or dermatologist will have the best recommendation for you. They know from patient feedback who does quality work and that's the only person you want.

LASERS

Everything is laser this and laser that. It seems to be one of the beauty buzzwords of this generation, and rightly so if it's the proper laser for the proper treatment. When it comes to facial hair removal, the verdict is not in on the laser. Data is limited on how long hair reduction lasts. Here's the scoop:

- Light-skinned patients with dark hair have the best results. The laser targets dark material.
- Blondes, redheads, and those with gray hair do not get as effective results.
- Those with darker skin tones must be careful of discoloration.
- Lasers are not the answer to facial peach fuzz.
- Be wary of quack claims: 0 percent regrowth, 100 percent hair removal, or permanent hair removal.

- There is a difference between laser and laser electrolysis. Only a professional can determine which treatment is for you. Laser electrolysis is not a blending of the two services.

- Check out the credentials of the person performing the laser service. Regulations differ in each state.

- Lasers usually get the best results on body (everything except the face) areas.

Hair in a Box

My career in the beauty business started at a small, wig salon in Los Angeles. Working part-time, I fit, cut, and styled wigs, wiglets, falls, and braids. I wore them, too. One day I was a redhead, another day a brunette. I stopped making the abrupt color changes when my nine-month-old son cried when I picked him up after work in my new burgundy shag.

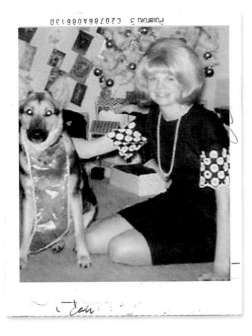

Remember the time the big head was in? I certainly wanted to be in, but perhaps I was so in I was out!

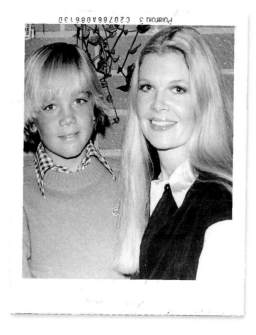

In the late seventies I finally learned the secret to natural-looking wigs. By using a little of your own hair in front, no one suspects that it's not your very own. My son kept my secret.

Today we are into natural hair that moves. Needless to say, many wig salons are out of business. The last time I was in a wig salon I helped my friend pick out a wig to cover her balding head from chemotherapy. It was a sobering experience. Yet, when she put on the right wig, she smiled that smile we all get when we like the way our hair looks. For many women, wigs and hairpieces are the solution to severe hair loss. The criterion is that they must look natural.

There are two types of wigs:

- *Handmade wigs* are the lightest and most comfortable but are more expensive because every hair is sewn on by hand.
- *Machine-made wigs* have wefts of fabric onto which are sewn strips of hair. The extra fabric makes them heavier and bulkier, but they cost less than handmade.

Wigs are made of two types of hair:

- *Human hair wigs* are real hair that is professionally colored to match your own. They can be quite pricey. Just like real hair, they need washing and styling.

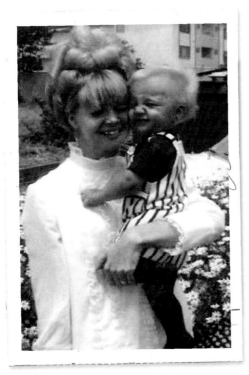

I never took it as an insult when people said "That's really a big hairpiece." Perhaps I should have.

- *Synthetic hair wigs* are made of artificial hair. It is prestyled but sensitive to heat. One steaming oven door opened in close range and you turn into a female Don King. Synthetic wigs have the advantage of being affordable and immune to the weather. On the negative side, they are a bit heavier.

Here's how you go about getting a wig that doesn't look like a wig:

- Find the best wig salon in your area. Hairdressers, cancer treatment centers, and friends who wear wigs are important references.
- Select a wig that looks like your hair in both style and color. This is not the time to make an abrupt change.
- Have the wig properly fitted. A wig that is too small looks like a cap. One that is too big screams "wig." If you have a small head, try one of the petite wigs.
- Once you select the right wig, have it fitted to your head. If the staff doesn't know how to fit a wig, find another salon. Very few people can wear a wig right out of the box. I don't know why, but they put about a third more hair in

wigs than any human can wear. Most thinning and cutting should be done on a wig stand with the final touches on you.

- Wear your wig right behind your natural hairline. The most common mistake is wearing a wig too far down on your forehead.
- Make sure it is comfortable. After it is on for ten minutes, you should be able to forget about it.
- Don't spray your wigs, let them blow in the wind. A stiff, sprayed head that doesn't move becomes a helmet.

Hair extensions are great if you want a quick fix of longer hair, but they are pricey, require maintenance, and damage your existing hair. For women of color they are a fantastic way to have long straight hair without chemical damage. For anyone with thin hair, they are not the best path to thicker hair.

HAIR FASHION MYTH: "WIGS LOOK WIGGY."

Not if they are the right ones. Many wigs are used on television and I dare you to guess by whom. A good wig, styled and fitted properly, is almost impossible to detect.

GROWN-UP GIRL'S HAIR RULE:

Hair is one of the grown-up girl's most important elements of appearance. It doesn't matter if your hair comes in a box, a transplanted hair shaft, or grows out of your own head. It only matters what the end result is. Good hair requires time and maintenance. The results are worth the effort. When you invest in your hair you invest in yourself. You are worth it.

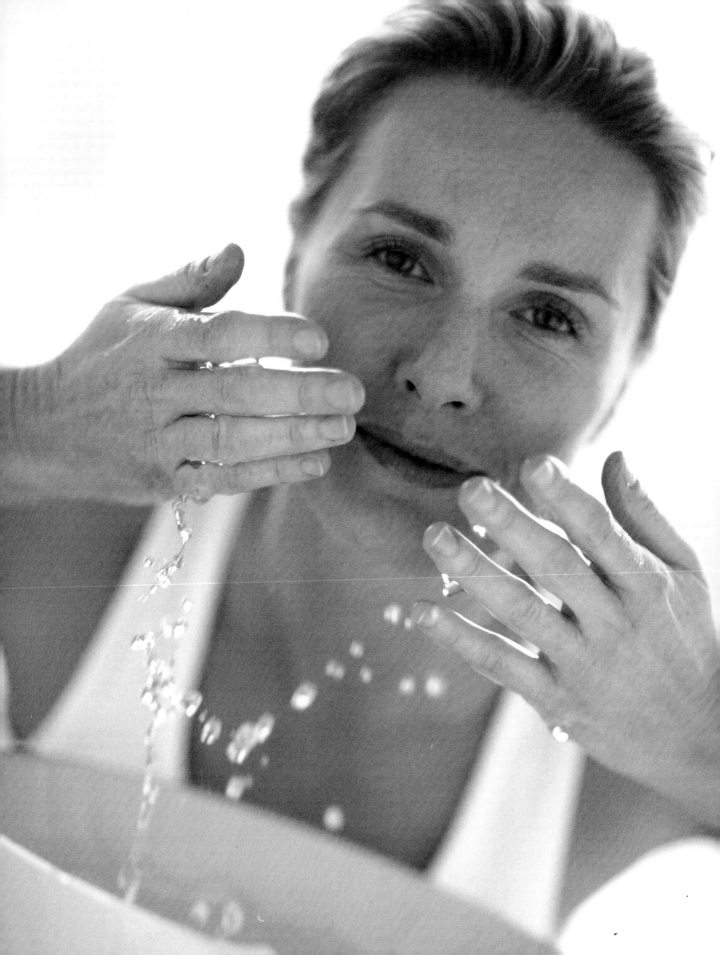

CHAPTER SIX

Skin

Today the focus is on healthy skin. We are past the era of heavy makeup concealment. We are in the age of skin care. While our mothers powdered, we want to glow—that Jennifer Aniston glow. Well, let's admit it, we also want her hair and her body. How does Jennifer get her look? It comes from a very important man in her life, a leading Beverly Hills cosmetic dermatologist and his recommended treatments and products.

I have interviewed the makeup artists who work on famous faces and even though they are mum about their clients' needs, they will say that they use very little makeup, only to enhance, not to cover. Today, it all begins with good skin.

Once you find the perfect skin care program for prevention, cleansing, and treatment your work is not done. You need to constantly adjust it along with any changes in your hormones, climate, or diet. The skirt length we wore in our twenties doesn't work in our forties. The skin care we practice in our thirties will not be the skin care we practice in our forties, fifties, sixties, or beyond. Our skin routines must evolve along with our beauty.

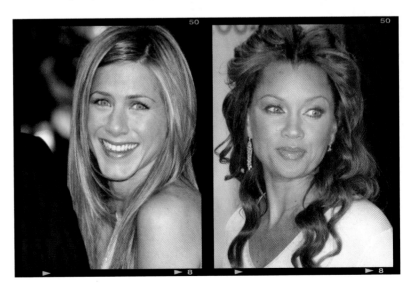

That Jennifer Aniston glow on the real deal.

That Jennifer glow on beautiful grown-up girl Vanessa Williams.

Banish Bad Habits

How do we get into bad habits? It's oh so easy. We simply repeat something that is often fun over and over without even being aware we are doing it and voilà—it's a habit. The myth "don't make an ugly face because your face might freeze" is somewhat true. All those squinting, laughing, and snarling expressions do indeed show up eventually on our faces. It's the repetition that causes the lines. It's the repetition of habits that causes sun damage, smoker's cough, and McDonald's burger thighs. I'm only interested in talking with you about the bad habits that concern your appearance and your health. Feel free to indulge in any others.

BAD HABIT #1 THE SUN

After all the years of hearing about sun damage, I finally got it. Of course I had to be hit over the head with brown spots on my chest and crepe paper texture on my neck. Somehow we never think it will happen to us.

How can we ever get it through our heads that the camel sheen sun glow that makes us look our absolute best will soon turn to crinkle that will make us look our worst. If you're not a sun worshiper, I applaud you. If you are, please stop immediately and try alternative tanning methods. If you were and you have reformed, read on, my fellow sun-damaged damsels.

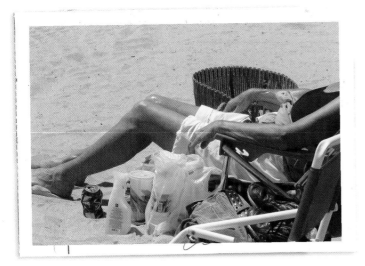

It looks relaxing and healthy. But when it comes to sun, looks can be deceiving.

How many times have we said or heard "Suntans make you look younger and healthier?" This is where we get into trouble. We look healthy, we feel healthy, and we bask in the compliments. But underneath that glow is the suntan truth: sun speeds up aging. Skin texture changes and I would be lying if I told you it changes for the better. Every year takes its toll on skin. That toll goes into overdrive with weather exposure.

Once the sun does its dirty little deed the continuation of tanning only makes the aging skin appear older. Many women actually feel that a tan hides wrinkles. It might hide brown spots, broken veins, and slightly diminish the appearance of cellulite, but wrinkles? It emphasizes them. Crinkles? It crinkles the crinkles. Skin texture? It becomes lizard texture. Now, we may want exotic animal skins on our bags and shoes, but not on our bodies. Bottom line, they may be golden brown, but they are still wrinkles exacerbated by sun.

Okay, so we did the damage and fried our bodies with baby oil and iodine and looked damn sexy with the results when we were twenty. Fortunately, at forty and beyond, we live in an age where products and technology are able to turn back the clock.

GROWN-UP GIRL'S ARTIFICIAL TANNING RULE:

Settle for looking less tanned. A little artificial tan goes a long way. A lot of artificial tan looks like what the name implies.

Is there a tanning product that goes on without streaking and looks natural? Do the tanning salons really work? Do artificial tans look good on mature skin? From a distance maybe, but up close? It's debatable. It all depends on how much tan you try to achieve and how well it is applied.

With home application, there usually are those telltale spots around the feet, knees, and elbows. I don't care how much preparation you do or how carefully you apply, self-tanning products still have not reached perfection. Are they better? Absolutely. But perfect? Not yet.

The younger the skin the better the self-tanning products look, simply because the skin is smoother. Older skin already has some issues that cause the tanning products to look even more artificial. The secret to good fake is light fake. Settle for a little color that looks almost natural rather than a lot of color that looks phony. The more color, the more emphasis on your skin's liabilities.

Is she actually trying to look like brown leather?

When applying self-tanners, go over any brown spots with a damp Q-tip. Change Q-tips often so you are removing the color from already pigmented spots rather than adding more. Time-consuming? Yes, but it beats tanning your brown spots. Remove those give-away dark streaks with a little nail polish remover on a soft tissue. Lightly, very lightly, whisk over the dark area until the color softens to match the rest of your self-tan. A heavy hand will give you a white streak.

BAD HABIT #2 SMOKING

When it comes to your health, it's hard to decide which is worse, the sun or cigarettes. The bottom line is the one you are more exposed to will cause the greatest harm. We once thought of the sun as healthy. We also thought of cigarette smoking as sexy. How the times have changed.

Read the warning label on the side of the cigarette package. Think of how you could apply the amount of money you spend yearly on cigarettes to products and services that make you look and feel better.

Yes, you can order dinner at the In-N-Out Burger drive-through window. Anyone who has ever bitten into one of their crunchy burgers will admit they are quite tasty. The old saying "you are what you eat" is actually quite truthful. Sometimes I really need to be a

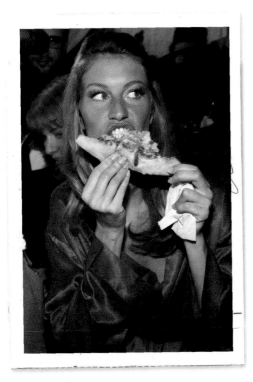

cheese pizza or a ballpark hot dog—and you do, too. Once in a while is not going to hurt you. What you put in does come out, in the tone of your skin, the cellulite on your body, and the width of your hips.

All the hyped low-fat, low-carb products may contain chemicals or an overabundance of sugar. The products that last forever in your fridge might remain in your body forever, too, in all the wrong places.

A young, ahead of his time agricultural student told me he made the switch to organic farming while earning his Ph.D. In class he was required to put on a protective suit (to spray a crop) that looked like he was fighting a chemical war. He only did that once. Are we putting those fruits and veggies into our bodies?

Organic food is more costly. You have to find a health food market in your neighborhood. The fruits and vegetables don't look as perfect. If we buy nonorganic produce are we paying for perfection and infection? Are we buying cancer? You can spend the time and money now, eating organic, or you can take the chance of spending it on treatments for disease at a later date.

Yes, even Gisele eats pizza, and then does the runway workout.

BAD HABIT #4 SMUSHING

We don't even realize some habits might be damaging. We think of sleeping as reenergizing. Someone even gave it the name "beauty sleep." But can beauty sleep really be aging sleep? Instead of rejuvenating our skin, are we wrinkling it?

Have you noticed that the deep facial lines and creases you wake up with in the morning now take a little longer to go away? Eventually they won't. Sleep on your back. Yes, it's harder and nothing beats cuddling your pillow. Silk pillows might make your hair last longer—if you're wearing 1980s hair—but they won't stop the smashed face.

BAD HABIT #5 FROWNIES

I trained in skin care and makeup with one of the former beauty industry legends, Miss Aida Grey. Her Beverly Hills salon was always filled with celebrities like Elizabeth Taylor, Cary Grant, Cher, Jacqueline Bisset, and Nancy Reagan. At that time Miss Grey was in her ageless sixties with the most beautiful skin I had ever seen on anyone, of any age. Every day she came to work with *Frownies* lifting up her eyebrows and cheek-bones. At first, you might think they were Band-Aids, but as you looked closer you realized they were little bits of adhesive designed to pull a wrinkle taut. They remained on until she prepared for her lunch date.

Once when she was teaching a plastic surgery client to cover her bruises, she looked the women squarely in the eyes and said, "Now you must learn to talk without expression to keep the wrinkles from returning." She was dead serious. Her philosophy was to move your face as little and as gently as possible with expressions, exercise, cleansing, and treatments.

I don't recommend we go around with stoic faces, or wear *Frownies* for hours on end. But she practiced what she preached, and she really did have stunning skin.

BAD HABIT #6 THE LAZY FACE

One of the most important things I learned from Miss Grey was that good skin requires work. The famous women who passed through her doors were living proof. On Academy Awards night, we worked from dawn to dusk, cleaning, treating, and making up the legendary faces of Hollywood.

Your skin doesn't care if you are rushed and must get out the door in the morning. It doesn't care if you have had a long and grueling day. It's greedy, and the older it gets, the greedier it becomes. It wants TLC all the time. If you have breakouts, change your wash-cloth, towel, and pillowcase daily. More laundry, but better skin.

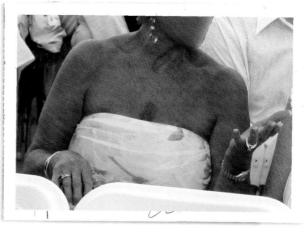

The price we pay for sun damage is most visible on the delicate skin of our chest. I say the price is way too expensive.

GROWN-UP GIRL'S SKIN HABITS RULE:

When it comes to your skin, you only get one. While you can't re-create a new skin, it's time to start repairing the one you have.

I would gladly trade my sun-damaged covering for a new one. At some point I am sure technology will come up with something that is close, but probably not for our generation. In the meantime, it's never too late to break your bad habits and replace them with good habits.

Quick Fixes

There are many makeup products on the market that claim "instant" gratification. When we look in the magnifying mirror on that overtired morning and wonder where the years went, we want that quick fix. But is anything really a quick fix?

It takes weeks to months to grow enough new cells to make wrinkles really better. Today there are hundreds of products on the market that claim to firm and plump wrinkles. The question is, do they do harm in the plumping? Dr. Mark Rubin, a leading cosmetic dermatologist in Beverly Hills says, "Many over-the-counter products that plump the skin contain low-level irritants. Any product that irritates enough to create minor swelling puts water in the skin, giving you a quick fix. It's not really making the wrinkles any better. It doesn't reduce the wrinkle, it temporarily changes the appearance of the wrinkle, but it's still the same old wrinkle. The cosmetic companies have to use some type of cheating ingredients to give the consumer that immediate gratification they crave. These products will only do so much. When you reach a plateau with over-the-counter remedies, a good doctor can take you to the next level in skin care."

GROWN-UP GIRL'S INSTANT RULE:
There is no such thing as "instant" skin care results.
Is instant anything ever as good as the real thing?

Spots and Dots

The freckles that once made you look young and healthy enlarge into age spots that beg for removal. That brown mole you think is a beauty mark might be an early indication of cancer if it has texture to the touch and seems to be growing. You need a good dermatologist to diagnose your spots and dots.

I am a spot-and-dot kind of girl, much to my dismay. I am paying the price for all those glorious hours in my canvas fold-up beach chair. Can I get rid of the evidence? Not completely, but along with my doctor I can keep it under control.

LIQUID NITROGEN

When I get this treatment, it reminds me of Halloween. The doctor comes in with a white Styrofoam cup with what looks like smoke coming out of it. He dabs the liquid nitrogen on my spots and dots and holds it in place for a minute. It stings a bit, turns a darker color, scabs over, and eventually fades. How much it fades depends on you. This is a good maintenance plan to do once a year before summer. The spots and dots never go away completely but they do become much less noticeable.

LASER

The photofacial is the laser used to treat sun damage. Its intense pulse light is attracted to pigment areas. It takes about five or six treatments to remove the spots, but you will see improvement after each one. They have made a big difference on my sun-damaged chest area. Use a numbing cream thirty minutes before your appointment. The laser feels like rubber bands being snapped against your skin. It's not painful, just slightly annoying. I am more annoyed with myself for all the time I spent in the sun in the first place.

CREAMS

There are over-the-counter and prescription creams for bleaching. The dilemma is how to prevent the damage from coming back. You can wear gloves everywhere. You can make sure every single inch of your body is totally covered with clothing. You can apply sunscreen on all exposed areas of your body three times a day and after every time you wash your hands—you get the gist. Whatever works for you becomes the right treatment.

Dr. Mark Rubin's Favorites

Here's an inside look at a prominent Beverly Hills cosmetic dermatologist's list of favorite skin care products.

Active cleansers with exfoliants to rejuvenate the skin surface and increase the penetration of other skin care products:

- Neutrogena Acne Wash (with Salicylic Acid)
- Aqua Glycolic Cleanser (with AHAs)

Moisturizers with wrinkle-reducing ability:

- Oil of Olay Regenerist

Collagen stimulators:

- Skin Medica TNS—a collection of growth factors that stimulate cell growth without dryness and peeling.

Rx:

- Avage—the newest antiaging retinoid, shown to work faster than Renova.

Body moisturizers:

- Eucerin Plus—a thicker-based moisturizer with alpha hydroxy acids to dissolve away the dead cells on the surface of the skin.
- Epionce Extreme Barrier Repair—a ceramide-based moisturizer that improves the skin's ability to retain water.

Pigmentation Rx:

- EpiQuin—a combination of retinol and hydroquinone. A very effective bleacher with the secondary benefit of rejuvenation from a vitamin A derivative.
- Glyquin XM with Sunscreen—a combination of alpha hydroxy acids, hydroquinone, and sunscreen in a very moisturizing base. This product is particularly good for patients with dry skin.

Lumps, Bumps, and Crevices

In the eighties, I am embarrassed to say, I actually provided cellulite wraps to my salon clients. The ace bandages were soaked in an Epsom salt and water solution. Their bodies were measured, logged, and marked before and after treatment. They were always smaller and a little smoother when the bandages came off, which was perfect when they needed to fit into a slim outfit. The caveat was that a few glasses of anything and they reverted back to their original size.

That about sums up the way I feel about cellulite treatments. Cellulite is caused by the accumulation of trapped fat and a lack of circulation to an area. I know dancers, athletes, and dedicated gym-goers who have cellulite. These are the lumps, bumps, and crevices of growing up.

Can you stop it? Can you improve the appearance of it? A little fake tan, a little kneading massage, a little anticellulite cream or body masque, and a lot of water might help, temporarily. I have tried them all and I simply don't feel they are worth the time and money. You know when it comes to appearance I am one who believes that time and money is well spent if it works. Some people are happy with the results of endermologie treatments, but then some people were happy with my ace bandage treatment. This is a machine that rolls, pulls, suctions, and massages the cellulite areas. If they worked as well as they claim we would not be a cellulite society. My personal opinion is that today's topical treatments don't eliminate the problem.

I am sure there will one day be a cure for cellulite and I hope it's within our lifetime. I will be the first in line. My guess is that it will be in the form of a pill. Cellulite is internal, so why shouldn't it be internally treated?

My clients were always happy with their cellulite wraps because they had instant gratification, and that was enough. If that's enough for you, spend your money. If not, try eating better, drinking more water, exercising more, and having robust massages of the rippled areas. These are as real as cellulite busters get.

Bottles and Jars

I have my favorite products as a professional and as a woman. I love to try anything new. It's that feeling you get when you open that jar or bottle of treatment that holds promise. Do I believe in miracles in bottle and jars? No, but I do believe that the right combination of products for your skin and body can make a difference. Just like finding the best in anything for your particular needs, you have to experiment. Talk with your friends, your cosmetician, and your doctors. Only you can determine what works for you. The thrill is in the hunt.

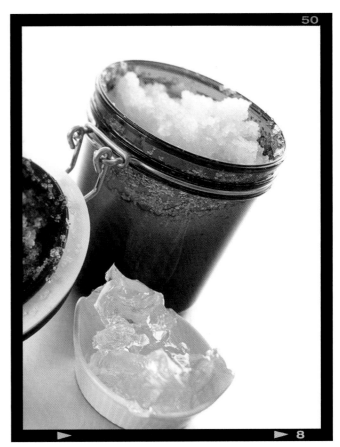

GROWN-UP GIRL'S PRODUCT RULE:
The bottom line is, if it works for you, it's the right thing.

Blemishes and Blotches

What does a grown-up girl do when she gets a pimple? Pimples, rashes, red blotches, and product irritations flare up at the most inconvenient time. Why is it when we want to look our very best our skin can sometimes have a mind of its own? The skin care labels promise everything and anything, and we willingly turn over our hard-earned money. So how do we determine what is the hype and what is the fact? We seek out professionals. A good dermatologist can zap your pimple, calm your rashes, and eliminate your blotches. A helpful pharmacist can guide you to good over-the-counter medical products. An informed cosmetic salesperson can assist you in the right product selection. If all else fails, a professional makeup artist can cover anything with the right application.

GROWN-UP GIRL'S TREATMENT RULE:

Treat your neck and chest as you do your face. Use those extra little dabs of moisturizer or creams for your earlobes. They need TLC just like the rest of us.

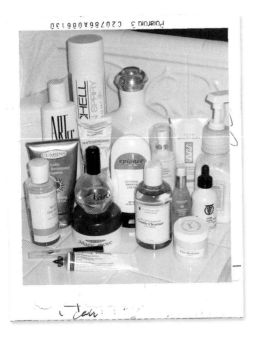

My bathroom countertop. Does it really take all these products to get me out the door? You betcha!

Matching

On my first visit to a cosmetic dermatologist I was greeted with "Your neck doesn't match your face!" Not "Hello, I'm Dr . . ." not "What can I do for you today?" This highly recommended celebrity doctor was only aghast that I didn't match. Insulted, I immediately found another doctor, only this time I asked him about the difference between the skin on my face and the skin on my neck. In my beauty routine I was spending all my time and effort on my face, never thinking that my neck deserved equal billing.

Of the billions spent on skin rejuvenating products, cosmetic dermatology, and plastic surgery, the majority of it is spent on the face. I was not alone. Once I became aware of the importance of matching I started to notice other mismatched women. The question that started to plague me is, why, when we take such care to make our faces look younger do we reveal chests, arms, or legs that have not had equal care? It doesn't matter how young your face looks if your body does not match.

While mixing vintage items with techie fabrics is considered high fashion in many circles, it's not when it relates to skin. Don't spend all your money on your face and let the rest remain untouched; either match or cover—just don't reveal. Why give our secrets away when we don't have to?

A Syringe of Promise

Cybill Shepherd claims she has had no plastic surgery. If that's true then she has been her cosmetic dermatologist's best patient. In a recent pictorial story on her, there is not a line or wrinkle to be found on her face. Mother Nature can't take a bow for that. Maybe the photo retoucher can?

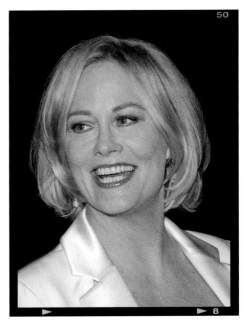

No plastic surgery???

What can we expect from cosmetic dermatology? Talking with leading Beverly Hills cosmetic dermatologist, Dr. Mark Rubin, I can assure you that we do live in the time of the ageless woman. This constantly changing and growing field of medicine has become the fountain of youth for our generation. Celebrities once traveled the world seeking the treatments that are now available in our neighborhoods. You can expect good results because a good doctor will deliver. Turning back the clock puts a dent in your pocketbook while it's putting a smile on your face. Before the treatment even takes effect, you feel like you have taken some control and it feels really, really good. Is this quest to look better an addiction? I think so, but what a healthy addiction to have. Pair this with regular exercise and healthy eating and you're matching your outside to your inside. If you're thinking this is way too self-indulgent, think again. We maintain our houses and cars. We maintain our gardens. Why shouldn't we maintain ourselves?

Here are some insights from Dr. Mark Rubin, Beverly Hills cosmetic dermatologist:

- Find the best cosmetic dermatologist by word of mouth. Ask your friends, plastic surgeons, even your hairdresser since they see and hear about a lot of "work."

- A good dermatologist will explain what you can and can't expect from any treatments. They will take an interest in you, not just the treatment.

- A good doctor will tell you when it's time for plastic surgery.

- You can now interrupt the aging process at any age.

- Depending on the treatment and your problem, you may be able to turn back the clock three to ten years.

- Injectable fillers and Botox are extremely safe products. You can stop at any time. No one burns a bridge if they use these new technologies. Most of today's treatments are very safe with minimal risk.

- Don't go for over-the-top results. Look natural. You know you've had too much Botox or fillers when your children start laughing at you. The honesty of the young is revealing.

- Skin of color has no problem with injectible treatments. But anything that irritates the skin or requires prolonged healing is sensitive to discoloration in the treated area.

- The basic difference between most over-the-counter products and products prescribed by your doctor are their strength and the delivery system.

- The topical products that make real overall changes in your skin's appearance are the products that don't show immediate results, but long-term improvement.

- It takes two to three weeks for a good treatment product to begin to show results, and at least three months to get the full benefits.

- There is no such thing as a safe tan. If you are getting any color from the sun, even with the strongest sunscreen, you are doing damage to your skin.

- Just because it's the latest therapy, doesn't mean it's the best therapy. Some of the treatments that get the most press may not live up to their hype. The press may say they are huge breakthroughs and quote doctors that also happen to be on the advisory boards of these companies while other doctors are returning the products or machines because they don't deliver what they promise.

- Are we coming to an age of treatments replacing surgery? That is the ultimate goal of cosmetic dermatology, but our current treatments are not there yet. You can stall the surgery while you keep ahead of the aging process.

High-Tech Faces

As good as the treatment and technology is, it is only as good as the person managing it. Once you have found the right doctor, you can try out the new cutting-edge treatments until you find the ones that work for you. It's the same with all types of medicine—you have to go through the test process to find the cures.

There might be areas of your face where Botox does the job, and then areas where you don't like the look. I love Botox on my neck. It eliminates the strained, bulging chords and firms up my jaw line. I didn't like Botox around my eyes. I just didn't feel or look like myself. I decided that I can live with a few eye crinkles. For many of you it might be just the opposite. Too much Botox can make you look frozen, and when you try to smile, you feel a strange sensation as if part of your face wants to stay put. Some people get headaches or flu symptoms for a short time after the injections. Others might get a little bruising at the injection site. I have had minor bruising, but it is easy to cover with makeup and disappears quickly. Watch some of the actors on the big screen. Whether crying, laughing, or angry, their faces never change expression. Why? Because they can't. Too much Botox is not a good thing. A little Botox here and there is a great thing.

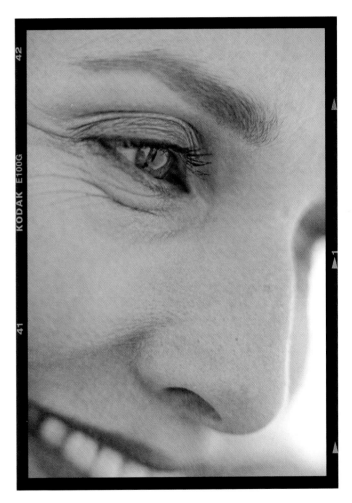

Fillers are amazing; they are also addictive. I never smoked, yet my mouth still had that smoker's pucker until I tried Restylane, one of the newest and most successful fillers. I have found nothing treats the creases around the sides of my mouth as well. I now will forgo a pair of shoes or maybe even a new bag for my Restylane injections. Does it hurt? If you had told me I would look forward to multiple shots around my mouth I would have thought you were crazy. But I do. By applying a numbing cream thirty minutes before my appointment and then icing the area before the injections, it really is not bad. The hardest part is when the doctor has to put his fingers in my mouth and squeeze the "putty" in place. So how do I get through the procedure? I think about how much better I will look when it's over. My vanity sets in and I barely notice the injections. The side effects and repercussions from Restylane can be a little swelling for up to forty-eight hours, a little inflammation and/or bruising at the injection site, and possible lumping or nodules. It's like silly putty plumping your skin out from the inside. I have never had any of these problems, but you need to be aware of the possibilities.

Temporary fillers are expensive because you have to re-plump every three to four months. A good doctor will adjust the type of filler to your needs. Once those heavy lines are plumped out they may just need a thin layer of filler to maintain. It may not cost less, but it looks best. I still always cringe as I pay my bill. But then I get home and over the next few days I see the difference. Do I look perfect? No. I look like a grown-up girl who maintains herself. I can rationalize and say it's because I work in television but the truth is I would do it even if I didn't. Fillers plump up areas that age depresses. No amount of makeup can hide the nasal folds that seem to get more pronounced each year. A little filler and they are gone. Instead of our faces sinking with age, they can retain that youthful fullness.

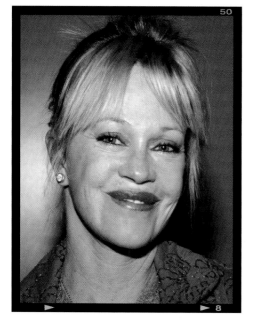

I know Melanie has a younger husband, but does she really think this is the way to keep up with him? Tip: never make your upper lip as big as your lower.

Are there permanent fillers? Data from Europe show that patients have had significant correction as long as ten to fifteen years after their injections with a product called Artecoil. This will be the first FDA approved permanent filler in America, under the name of Artefill. It's made up of microscopic beads of PMMA (polymethylmethacrylate) suspended in a matrix of bovine collagen. The U.S. product will be the improved version with smaller, more uniform beads of PMMA. At the time of injection there is immediate correction because of the collagen. The body responds to the PMMA beads by encapsulating them in new collagen growth. This creates more volume in the skin, so, as the injected collagen is absorbed, it is replaced by the body's own collagen. My recommendation is to try the temporary filler first, and make sure you like both the look and the doctor. It's always better to ease into anything permanent.

Be sure that you don't go overboard with a good thing. We don't want that rounded baby face look even though it means no wrinkles. We don't want Angelina Jolie lips just because they look sexy on her. There are way too many oversized lips walking around and I can't help but think they feel they are getting their money's worth by adding more. The best spent cosmetic money is in the subtle results. Don't go for that extra bit of filler that takes you over the edge to fake. We don't want to be Stepford Wives or Desperate Housewives. Be realistic. Be sure you find a good and gentle doctor. It's essential to first do a patch test for allergies. There are quite a few filler products on the market. Good doctors will use different types and textures of fillers for different areas.

Mini-peels, lunchtime peels, glycolic peels, and facials are high-tech treatments when you have them at the dermatologist office. They will cost more than in salons but the results are usually better simply because the strength of the products are stronger. Are they worthwhile? If you get results, yes. I find what I call the "lightweight" treatments are exactly that. You get instant results. If you do a series you get better results.

THE GROWN-UP GIRL'S GUIDE TO STYLE

The caveat is once you stop, so do your results. It's all a matter of how much money and time you have to invest. For an important event they are fantastic. For everyday they are expensive, but if they work for you in both aesthetics and budget, you get to make the decision.

The high-tech machines that eliminate sun damage, enlarged pores, and fine lines are definitely worth a try. Removal of the aging tiny veins on your legs is just an injection or zap away. Threading mini face-lifts and acupuncture facial treatments are just a few options available to our generation. The technology is changing so rapidly that every year brings more age-defying treatments. We are all individuals, with our own expectations and goals. What I do promise you is that there are professional treatments and solutions for almost every issue you have.

When I told my dermatologist about this book and that I was going to tell the truth about everything to do with maintenance, his comment was "Well, I hope you're not going to be one of those who go on TV and deny they have done anything." How true. I love it when some well maintained woman goes before the cameras and denies that she does anything to her face, or concedes that she has had a mini eye lift, when in reality everyone in the business knows she is the result of all that's available.

If you are comfortable with the way you look naturally, that's wonderful. If you are looking for change-of-life explanations, go to a shrink. If you simply want to look better, go for it. The treatments that are available now are truly incredible. If you are in doubt, just look at the celebrities on the red carpet. They might not admit to what they are doing, but I guarantee you, they are doing something.

Are you intrigued by the Botox parties? Don't be. True, it will be a professional giving the Botox, but at what strength? Perhaps just enough to get you hooked instead of the amount you would get in a doctor's office. Be leery of home parties that claim to do what to date has only been offered in doctor's offices. Be very leery. Don't mix social gatherings and medical procedures. Pedicure and Botox in one quick stop at your local beauty salon? Forget it. You want to go to your salon for salon treatments. Anything with a needle or a laser is a medical treatment. I say, stay very far away from any doctor who would consider high-tech group treatments or multitasking beauty salons trying to be more than they should.

Making the Cut

What are we looking for when we decide to have plastic surgery? To look better? Absolutely. To feel better? It goes without saying. To be perfect? If you are going into plastic surgery for perfection I seriously think you need to take a gigantic step back. I am an advocate of doing a little maintenance at a time. The twelve-hour surgeries to do your nose, chin implant, and face-lift can leave you looking like someone else. I say look like your very best self. If your eyes are puffy, consider having them done. If your neck is sagging, get a little tightening. If your cheekbones are dropping, try a little lifting. Make subtle changes.

Why does everyone on television look so ageless? Because they know the secret of ongoing maintenance. They take a small vacation and tweak a bit here; "on assignment" may mean a little tweak there. This way they return looking like they went on vacation, not like they had plastic surgery. Movie stars go in for fine-tuning before a big movie or awards program. Have you ever seen a female star at a media function looking anything other than perfect? Have you ever seen a wrinkle on the red carpet? Who can handle the wrath of the media? Remember, they are the professionals. Their perfection is not good genes as many claim. It's not the latest holistic diet, and it's certainly not facial exercises. That perfection most likely comes as a result of a scalpel, syringe, or laser. What celebrities spend and do to maintain themselves is beyond the average woman's comprehension.

Once you have a good experience with plastic surgery (and they should all be good experiences if you do your preliminary homework), you realize why people go back for more. The majority of facial cosmetic surgery is relatively painless. It may be uncomfortable and a little scary looking during the healing process, but pain? Give me the plastic surgeon for face work over the dentist drilling any day. The results are addictive.

When it comes to body surgery, I personally would rather exercise my body to whatever shape I can attain rather than have surgery. But I know of many women who have had body procedures done and are delighted with the results. My concern is that some people feel it's an instant diet, a permission slip to eat whatever you want. Any body surgery must be considered a part of your maintenance, not your total maintenance. While our faces heal the fastest, bodies can sometimes take longer and be more painful in the recuperation process. Liposuction requires kneading after the surgery to increase the results and this is quite painful. Can you imagine someone firmly kneading your body after an operation? The thought makes me hurt. Tummy tucks are in a very sensitive area that can cause discomfort. Yet, the plastic surgeons' offices are busier than ever with body work. I have friends who say that body surgery is a breeze and others that say it is excruciating (but then, I have friends who don't mind the dentist either). Your pain threshold, the amount of surgery you're getting, and your physical condition will all contribute to your pain level and your healing time. Very few people who have one elective surgical procedure stop at that. Over 50 percent of the women that have plastic surgery come back for an encore. Just as in theater encores, it's better to leave, or in this case stop, when you are ahead.

There comes a time when you can start looking like you are desperate to hold on to your youth. Dyan Cannon has an incredible figure and that fabulous long curly blonde hair and yet when I see her at the Laker games I can't help but think she has gone too far with her face. It's such a beautiful face that now looks a little too distorted and desperate to me. Stop while you are ahead. Stop while you look great for whatever age you are, not the age you wish you were.

How do you know when it's time for surgery?

- You start to focus on one area of your face instead of your overall look.

- No matter how much eye shadow you put on, you still look tired.

- You start spending an inordinate amount of money on treatment creams. Save your money, even the most expensive creams do not take the place of surgery.

- You keep changing your makeup, hairstyle, and clothing looking for some way to look better.

- You tear up those close-up photos before anyone can see them.

- You have lost the majority of your breast tissue from nursing and hormonal changes.

- You are simply unhappy with how you are aging.

Dr. Gary Tearston is a Beverly Hills plastic surgeon who practices at Cedars-Sinai Medical Center. He is held in high regard by both his peers and his patients. His office is always a beehive of activity of people all ages. Trying to get him to sit down for an interview is almost impossible. In this town where there are hundreds of choices, he's worth waiting for.

Here is Dr. Tearston's plastic surgery maintenance program for women who are forty-plus. Maintenance should begin in your twenties and thirties with protection from the sun and avoidance of smoking.

THE FORTIES:

- The first signs of aging are in the eyelids with puffiness and or loose skin.

- Resurfacing of the skin can be done for sun damage.

- If you are a squinter or a frowner (usually those with light skin and eyes), you may want your eyebrows raised.

- Some women need a little tightening of their jowl and neck.

- 60 percent to 70 percent of women could benefit from a face-lift to tighten loose skin.

- Almost everyone can benefit from a face-lift at this age. If you have already had one it might need a little tightening.

- Fillers and Botox work well in addition to surgery. The questions are the length of time they last. Many claim to last far longer than is realistic.

- It's time to stop surgery when you can't be helped in the way you think you can. Pulling and tightening is only for substantial looseness of the tissue. You may also need filling and resurfacing. Don't get confused between wrinkles and looseness. Pulling your skin tight to see what results will look like is not an accurate test if there are wrinkles and not significant looseness. When there is not a significant looseness to begin with surgery will look distorted.

WATCH OUT FOR THESE GIMMICKS:

- Expensive little ways to improve yourself without surgery. Most have yet to be proven. I haven't been impressed with many of them. If you have lots of money and trust someone, fine, just don't expect any great improvement. These include thermage and cool lasers that are designed to heat the deeper collagen layers. Results are highly unpredictable and the science questionable. They need large double-blind studies and less advertising.

- Anything that promises too much too quickly. I would advise you to read Hans Christian Andersen's "The Emperor's New Clothes."

Dr. Tim Miller, head of plastic surgery for the UCLA Medical Center says, "Cosmetic dermatology will never replace plastic surgery. They are two separate issues. Cosmetic dermatology is an adjunct, not a replacement, to plastic surgery. Nothing can replace a face-lift." Here are Dr. Miller's recommendations if you're considering plastic surgery:

- Consult with several doctors. Do they seem honest, trustworthy, and credible? Are their offices neat and orderly? Ask to see before and after photos and talk to some of their patients. Eye, ear, nose, and throat doctors are good for surgery in the areas they are trained in, but not for full face-lifts.

- Make sure the surgeon goes over what is going to happen and answers *all* of your questions before surgery. Unhappy patients are ones who have unrealistic expectations.

- Be leery of practices that advertise miracles. They attract patients who want quick fixes.

- It's never too late to have surgery as long as you are healthy. Health is the main issue, and this is real surgery. Doctors are making an incision with a knife, in an operating room with anesthesia. There are risks and complications even though they are extraordinarily low. You are dealing with a knife. It's not a beauty parlor; it's not an injection.

- Don't have the "might as well get it all done at once" attitude. As you go into different areas on the body the risks go up. You are asking a lot of the body to do healing in different locations. Extreme makeovers entail too much concentration and endurance for the surgeon and for the patient.

- Liposuction is the most popular cosmetic surgery. The secret is your skin tone. Good skin tone will contract after the fat is removed. Lipo is not a weight loss solution. What it does very well is improve the contour in areas that tend to accumulate fat that is dimpled: upper thighs, inner thighs, knees, abdomen, and under the chin and neck. If you are looking for an overall reduction in your size, lipo is not for you.

- The latest technique is not always the best. Women's magazines and TV doctors talk about the latest, the hottest, and the exciting variations. There are not really that many ways of doing a face-lift. If it's a big departure from an existing standard, you have to ask yourself, do you want to be the first in line?

- Be consistent to your age. The face needs to match the body. Cosmetic surgery is not an age-related procedure; it needs to make you look better, not a certain age. Age is not determined only by your facial appearance. You are still the chronological age you are, but you can always improve it. Look great at your age, but look like yourself—that's who you are.

GROWN-UP GIRL'S AGING RULE:

Don't try to look like anyone other than your best self.

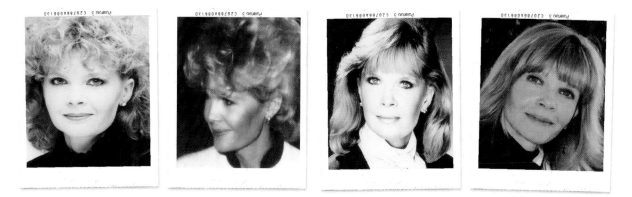

Yes, they are all me, spanning from the '80s to today. You can see the results of my maintenance programs and of course my evolving hairstyles.

Cosmetic dermatology treatments now allow us to turn back the clock without surgery. They are amazing, and they are expensive. You have to weigh their value. You have to know when to start and when to stop. You want the best of what's available, not the most. Cosmetic dermatology and plastic surgery can indeed keep us ageless. The question we must ask is, how far is far enough?

Christine's Maintenance

- **Nip:** In my early forties, for a major crease between my eyes. I was tired of looking angry. It was a breeze, no wonder everyone is doing it.

- **Tuck:** A few years later for my upper and lower lids. I knew it was time when I started using darker and darker eye shadow to define my eyes. Downtime was minimal, it was easy to hide the bruises with stylish sunglasses.

- **Nip:** A few years later to make my neck match the rest of me; instant jawline.

- **Burn:** Laser peel on my upper lip, to remove "smokers wrinkles" (and I never smoked). Don't sit across from your husband while healing . . . it's not pretty.

- **Burn again:** Such good results on my upper lip I decide my whole face needs a little peel. Ouch! This one was tough. My skin glows, but I'll never do it again.

- **Tuck:** My lower lids. Where does all that puffy stuff keep coming from?

- **Inject:** My new maintenance plan, a little Restylane here, a little Botox there.

The Instant Diet?

Liposuction's a lot more costly than the latest diet book and a lot more serious. My theory is that it should only be for those who are at their ideal weight, have a regular workout routine, and eat healthy diets, but still possess patches of fat around the tummy, thighs, knees, and upper arms. It is not an instant diet. It does not replace taking care of your body. It is not an alternative, it is the final tweaking. If you are disciplined about your body and just can't exercise away those saddlebags, or your three pregnancies left you with a roll of unwanted inner tube padding around your middle that no amount of exercise or diet will remove, then go for it. If you are looking to munch on tortilla chips and Snickers bars (it makes me yearn just writing about them) while you watch your nightly TV, don't waste your money. Will you look better? Yes! Will you get tons of compliments? More than tons. Will you feel better? Like you conquered the world. Will it last? Not if you don't change your unhealthy lifestyle. You might as well spend that money on chips, Snickers, and rented movies.

Technology is available to sculpt your body into that celebrity shape. Many celebs do and many of us lust to look like them. They have unlimited money and time and must compete with the new generation of stars on an ongoing basis. Can you even imagine having a career with so little security? It makes that nine-to-five job look a little sweeter. So when is body surgery right for the rest of us?

- When the best of the support bras no longer supports.

- When that once voluptuous bosom gives you major back problems, not to mention makes you look ten pounds heavier.

- When no amount of diet or exercise will remove the fat pads on your body or the inner tube around your waist.

- When you have maintained your weight with a healthy diet and exercise and can't get rid of all that excess loose skin.

Remember that the treatment is only as good as the hands that are performing it. Make sure you are in the very best hands. Having any elective surgery is a very important decision. It's one of the only surgeries where we get to make many decisions. Don't treat it lightly. Do your homework. Make sure this is what you want. Be realistic about expectations. Don't try to change your life or dramatically alter your look. Plastic surgery should be to enhance what you have, not change who you are.

Chiclets

The very first maintenance procedure I did was bonding my teeth. I spent all my teenage years hiding my "fang" tooth. The reality is that you can't hide your teeth, you have to fix them.

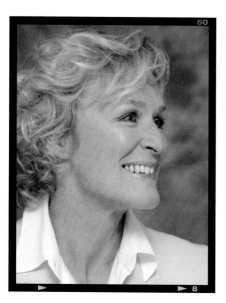

My stepdaughter never smiled in photographs, ever. When she was planning her wedding she decided to bond her teeth. Her fiancé agreed with us that it seemed so unnecessary. She didn't. She always yearned for what she called "Chiclets" teeth. So she did the research, made the appointments, paid her money, and had it done. The wedding photos came back and there was her smile, one we had never seen in pictures before and she looked truly beautiful. While it didn't seem important to other people, it was very important to her. That's what beauty procedures are all about. Only you can make the decision on what's right for you.

A pretty smile is always beautiful, on many levels. Crooked, dingy teeth are never attractive, regardless of the perfect outfit, a great hairdo, and glowing makeup. I would place cosmetic dentistry at the top of anyone's maintenance list.

Glenn Close has that perfect "Chiclets" smile.

Cosmetic Dentistry

Dr. Larry Rosenthal is one of the leading cosmetic dentists in New York City. He has transformed dentistry into artistry. Here are his recommendations.

Corrective smiles:

- Sit in front of a mirror and talk or read out loud. Look at what you see or have someone take your picture. This is what others see as you talk. Look at the bottom teeth as well as the uppers. Many people only concentrate on the upper teeth. You see the upper teeth when you smile and the lower teeth when you talk.

- As you age you see less teeth and less lips. That can now be corrected.

- Get a professional consultation before you try anything.

- Ask your doctor for a computer simulation. This will show you what you will look like when the work is done.

- Try Invisalign braces. They are so clear no one can tell you have them. It is never too late to wear braces.

- Veneers are half as thin as they were ten years ago and twice as strong.
- You can have laser surgery to improve your gum line. No more scalpels and sutures. It is almost painless, heals almost instantly.

Over-the-counter whiteners:

- Most products are somewhat effective for most of the population.
- Night White bleaching.
- Super Smile.
- White strips (if you can keep them in place).
- Peroxyl mouthwash by Colgate. Kills bacteria and maintains whitening.
- Toothpastes don't stay on the teeth long enough to whiten.

Professional treatments:

- Bleach trays, available in different strengths with prescription for at-home use. Stronger strengths for day, for shorter time spans. Weaker strengths for night because of longer time use. Don't be a bleach junkie. Overbleaching may weaken your teeth and they will take on a gray translucent color, not the color of choice.
- Zoom Laser System—the best office treatment with the least amount of sensitivity. One hour can lighten up to twenty teeth.
- Often a combination of laser and bleach tray treatment will get the maximum results.

My sister invested a small fortune in the bonding of her teeth, and after quite a few years they are still amazingly white. Her secret is clear liquids. She exchanged red wine for white, diet coke for sparkling water. Any liquids with color can also color your teeth and bonded teeth don't respond to bleaching products or treatments. So if you want to maintain white bonded teeth, think clear drinks.

Naked Nails

We can't forget our nails. It doesn't matter how incredible your outfit looks if your nails are broken and chipped. It doesn't matter how much you paid for your designer shoes if your toenails are unkempt.

I feel one of the biggest age revealers are a woman's hands. My family history is veined hands. I hide mine a lot. I admit when it comes to pampering mine I am not as disciplined as I should be. Are you? Do we always use rubber gloves? Apply lotion after every household chore involving water? Apply sunscreen daily? Probably not. Should we? Who has the time or inclination? And so we live with the life story that our hands are determined to tell.

If your hands don't pass inspection, try these tips:

- Keep your nails short and naked, or nearly so. Almost nothing is more dated than long, fake, colorful fingernails.

- Go for short, natural squarish-shaped nails. Anything that even resembles a point screams "time warp." Stop the screaming. Choose polish colors that are translucent and natural: barely-there blush colors, pale nude to soft pink tones, clear, or a natural looking French manicure.

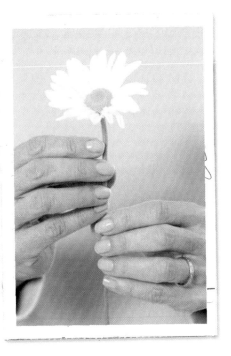

These are well-groomed nails that don't draw attention. Who wants to be known for their fingernails?

- No iridescent sparkle, multiple layers of lacquer, or decorations (please!), no gemstones, no false nails, gel nails, or extensions of any kind. I don't care what the latest nail trend is, resist it.

- Pass those over-the-top rings on in your family or reset them into subtle bands or beautiful brooches. The bigger the diamonds, the more attention you gather and once they get over the size of your bling, there are those hands again, giving away your secrets.

- Gloves are the best cover-up, but you need to have the situation warrant them.

- Try keeping your palms up when your hands are in resting mode. Palms have been shielded from the sun and wear and tear. And talking? Just keep them exquisitely calm in your lap while others are flinging theirs about.

- Apply cuticle oil when you start your makeup routine every day; multitask to your benefit.

- If your bag is not too heavy, add a good moisturizing hand cream with sunscreen—it's never too late—and try to use it every time you apply your lipstick.

- Don't forget those toenails! Keep them short and simple. French manicures are a bit much for my taste on toes; they never look natural. A nice nude color blends if you have feet issues. If your toes are looking pretty good, a hot pink, burnt orange, or clear red can be very sexy. Just like your fingernails, don't add any sparkle, paintings, or gimmicks.

NAIL MYTH: "LONG, BEAUTIFUL NAILS ARE THE SIGN OF A LADY." LONG NAILS, EVEN IF BEAUTIFUL, ARE THE SIGN OF A TIME-WARPED GROWN-UP GIRL.

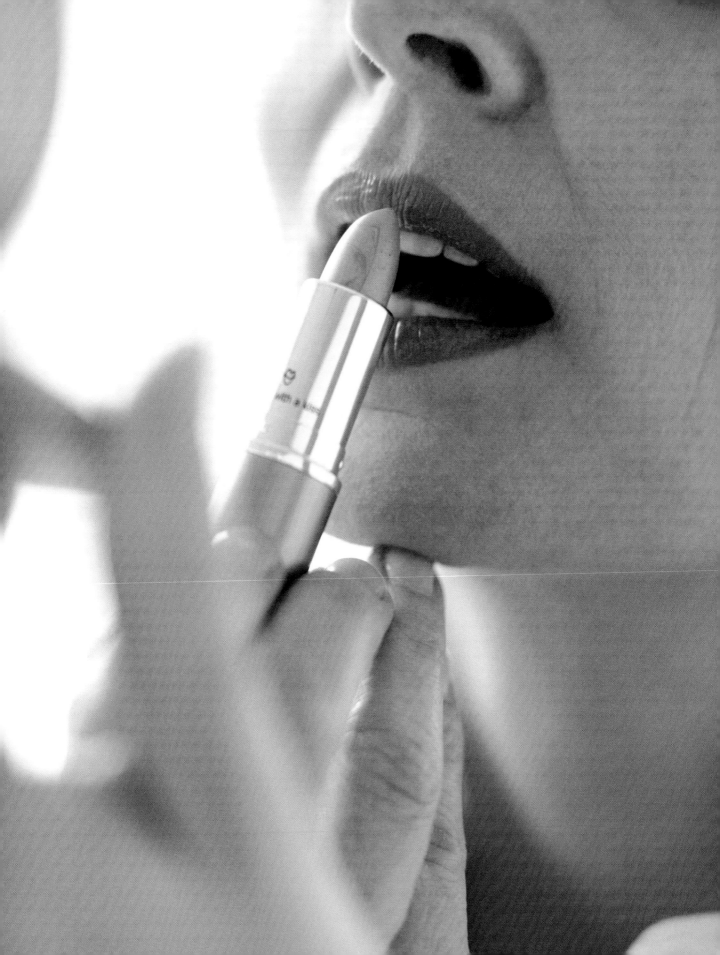

CHAPTER SEVEN

Makeup

I learned about makeup from my mom. I would sit on the floor and watch her at her vanity table putting on her daily "face." As a teenager I spent hours in the bathroom trying to re-create the cover girl's makeup in the latest edition of *Seventeen* magazine. At twenty-four I landed my first job applying makeup professionally. I felt like I was getting paid to play. I have never lost my passion for makeup. I am a true believer in its magic. Like my mom, I try never to go out of the house without putting on my "face." It makes me feel better about myself.

Makeup is our best friend. After teaching thousands of women to apply their makeup, I know firsthand that it is a skill anyone can learn. For the forty-plus woman it's about wearing makeup that doesn't look made up. We don't need to wear the trends, we need to wear what flatters. We don't need to make statements with our makeup, we need to make our statements with our entire look. Makeup is a key element to that look.

Tubes, Tubs, and Pots

As young as you may feel, a little eyeliner and lipstick can make you feel even younger. It's simply that magic in a tube, tub, or pot. It can be our biggest ally (think of Lauren Hutton and Michelle Pfeiffer with their freshly scrubbed, yet subtly made-up faces), or our worst enemy (think of Jackie Collins still wearing her '80s makeup masque). Makeup styles change and, just as with fashion, we must evolve with them: adapting what is appropriate, eliminating what is not, and simplifying our routine. We don't need more makeup products, we need fewer, but we need the right ones. Forget the fads, it's time to strive for subtle. No harsh makeup, just hidden enhancers that enable us to present our face every day in its absolute best way.

It's time to clean out our drawers. How do we decide what to keep, what to toss? I have the inside scoop on what does and doesn't work: no fake promises, no exaggerated claims, no gift with purchase specials, just good sound advice.

Makeup: What to Keep and What to Toss

Toss:

- Makeup you haven't worn in a year
- Products with too much sparkle or shine
- Eye shadows that scream "color"
- Mascara that requires more than two coats
- Heavy, opaque foundations
- Dark or overly bright lip liner pencils
- Any makeup your teenagers are begging for—if they want it you probably don't

Keep:

- Flat powder eye shadows in subdued colors
- Cake eyeliners in covered containers
- Eye and lip pencils in soft colors
- Sheer foundations and tinted moisturizers with SPF 15 or higher
- Your favorite lipsticks—if you love 'em, then keep 'em

The Primpers

THE DAYTIME BASIC FACE

This is my favorite everyday makeup. You can adjust it to fit your needs. It works for almost everyone, regardless of color or age. It shouldn't take you more than ten minutes to apply. Remember, you don't want it to look like you tried too hard.

1. Skin treatment

If you need a pore minimizer, a neck cream, or a hydrating cream, apply them first. Use treatments lightly and only on the necessary areas. Noses almost never need added lubricants. Let treatments dry while you complete the next step.

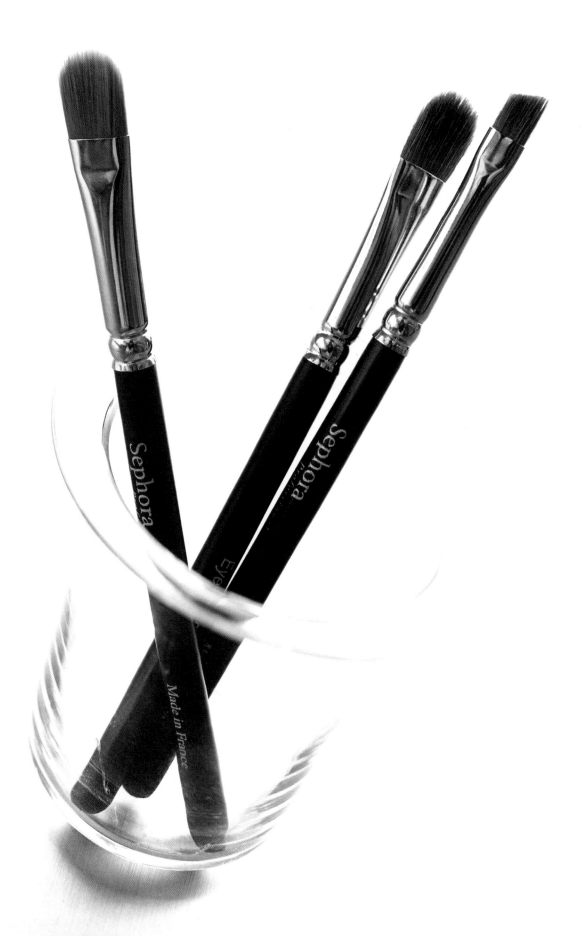

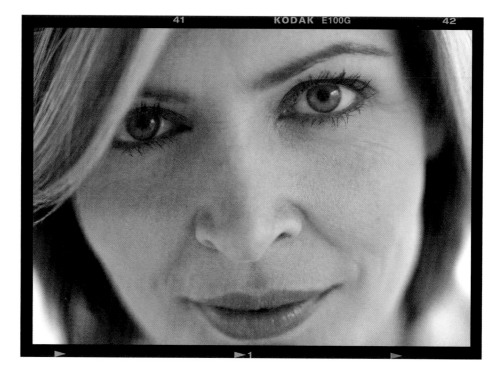

2. Brows

With magnifying glasses, a magnifying mirror, and bright sunlight, check for any stray hairs and tweeze them away. If you can't get a hair on the first few pulls, give it a day and it will come out easily. Which is worse, a hint of a hair or a gap in your skin? If you have your brows professionally shaped you still need a daily check. Fill in with color as needed, always keeping both color and shape natural.

3. Moisturizer

If you are using a tinted moisturizer, apply in step 8. If you will be wearing a foundation, apply a moisturizer with sunscreen now. Let it dry.

4. Lashes

Curl your lashes without phone calls or distractions. Lashes need to remain on your lids, not in the curler.

5. Eye shadow

If you like a little lid color, add it now. The key word is little. Powders should be neutral colors, without sparkle. Keep the majority of your shadow close to your eyelash line; no sharp wings or points. For a more natural look, use a powder eyelid base color to even out your skin tone.

No fake sparkle around your eyes. Make the sparkle come from the inside.

6. Eyeliner

I recommend the dry, cake liners that you apply with a damp brush. They stay on longer. If liner pens, pencils, or liquids work best for you, stick with them. Apply eyeliner in between your lash line by holding up the upper eyelid. Then apply above the lash line on the top lid. Always, always smudge the top of the line with either a damp brush or a dry Q-tip. For more definition, lightly line the lower lashes. For a fresh daytime look, use only mascara on the lower lashes. Heavy lines on the lower lashes can drag the eye down.

7. Spots and dots

Dot a little *concealer on any problem areas*

8. Foundation or tinted moisturizer with sunscreen

Foundation or tints must, must, must match your skin tone on both your neck and face. Check in bright daylight. Apply lightly. Any collecting in creases or lines will emphasize them. Blend off any excess with a clean makeup sponge. Never apply to your neck.

9. Mascara

Apply to your upper and lower lashes. Don't try to put all your mascara on in one coat. Let it dry and then reapply. Allow any mascara smudge to dry and then remove with a dry Q-tip; only wet mascara smears.

10. Enhancer eyeliner

A little brown, navy, charcoal, or aubergine powdered eye shadow can enhance your liner if you apply it right on top. It also softens your liner and holds it in place. Add a little more thickness to the outer corners of the eye for stronger definition.

11. Eye concealer

With a firm small brush, apply concealer in the inner corner of the eyes and on any spots, dots, and dark areas on your face that are still showing. Blend the edges gently with a clean Q-tip or finger. Never use concealer under the entire eye, only where needed for darkness and discoloration.

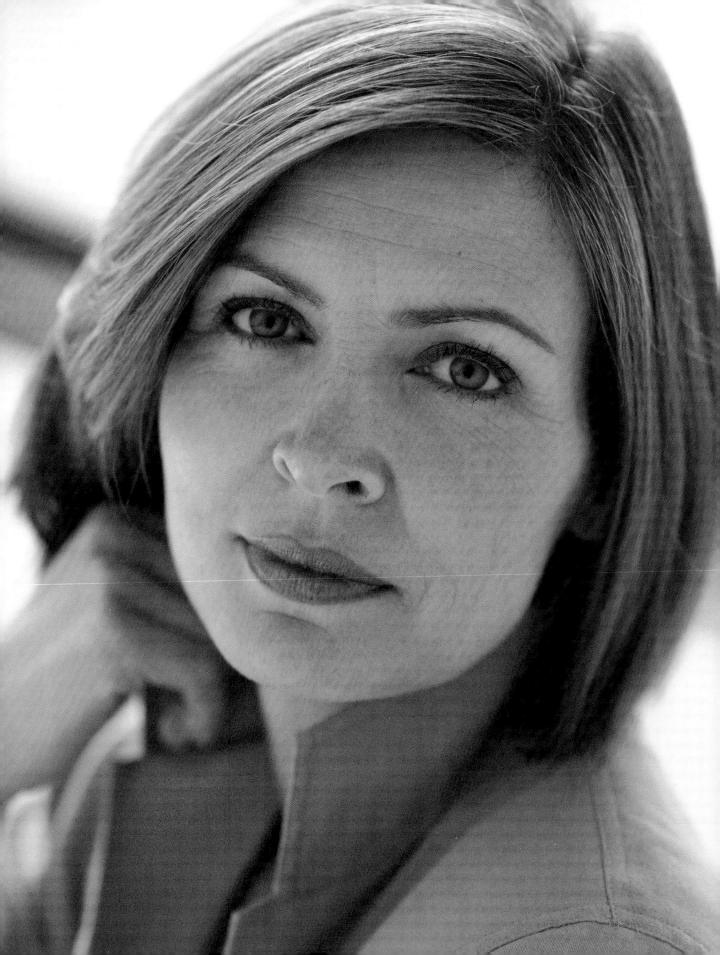

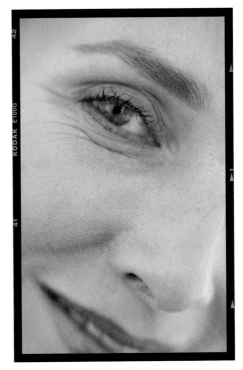

GROWN-UP GIRL'S BLUSHER RULE:

Less is best.

12. Base blush

*This is your overall cheek blush. It should be on the more
neutral side: darker than your skin tone without being too
colorful. This defines your cheekbones.*

13. Enhancer blush

*This is a slightly brighter color used only on the apples of the
cheeks. Blend both base and enhancer blush with a blending
spatula. I find it almost impossible to get the right amount of
color without looking artificial with only one color of blush.*

14. Lip treatment

*Plumpers, fillers, or even good old ChapStick. Anything that makes your lips look
naturally softer, moister, and maybe a tad larger.*

15. Lipliner

*A pencil in a nude color. You don't have to match your lipliner to your lipstick. It
racks up more sales for the beauty companies but it looks like you lined your lips.
The goal is to sneak in a bit of extra lip and keep your lip color on longer.*

16. Lipstick or gloss

Your favorite colors or shines. Blot to prevent lipstick on teeth.

17. Pass muster

*The final and most important test is to remove your magnifying glasses and mir-
ror and look at your overall face in bright daylight. Nine times out of ten a little
blending will be required. Sometimes you need a little more blush or eyeliner.
Sometimes, a little less. This is the way your daily world will see you. Is it the way
you want to be seen?*

Paint Box

Our drawers might look like a paint box of colors. Our faces must look like a restrained blending of tones. Here are the products and colors you will find in my dressing table drawers:

Foundation

- Daytime: I like to keep it light and natural with Laura Mercier's foundation primer and tinted moisturizer with SPF 20.

- Nighttime: I still like to keep it natural with Vincent Longo's water canvas primer and creme-to-powder foundation.

- Cover-up: I dot Laura Mercier's camouflage compact on any blemishes, red spots, or discoloration marks. It's amazing.

- Under eyes: I have used Yves Saint Laurent's Touché Éclat for years and love its lightness. It never cakes.

Blush

- My basic summer blush color is Clé de Peau's powder bronzer, used very lightly. I like the hint of sunglow.

- My spring, winter, and fall blush color for day is Fresh's Age of Innocence cream blush. It's a soft pink. I dust Benefit's Dandelion Blush over my basic blush all year long for a very soft pink, barely there color. For a peachier look I use Benefit's Georgia Blush on top. Sometimes I mix the peach and the pink together. I feel you need to vary your blush depending on your skin tone that day. Sometimes we need a little more, sometimes a little less. For night, I like Vincent Longo Mocha Crème blush because it's a little deeper. Then I add a little of Bobbi Brown's Sand Pink for a little more color, a little more definition.

Mascara

- I have tried them all and keep going back to Estee Lauder's More Than Mascara in black. It stays in place all day and night and so do my eyelashes.

Eye liner

- Makeup Forever's Cake Eyeliner in brown. Sometimes, I venture into a navy or gray and when I'm adventurous a dark brick color. This liner does not smudge, ever, unless you see a heart-wrenching movie.

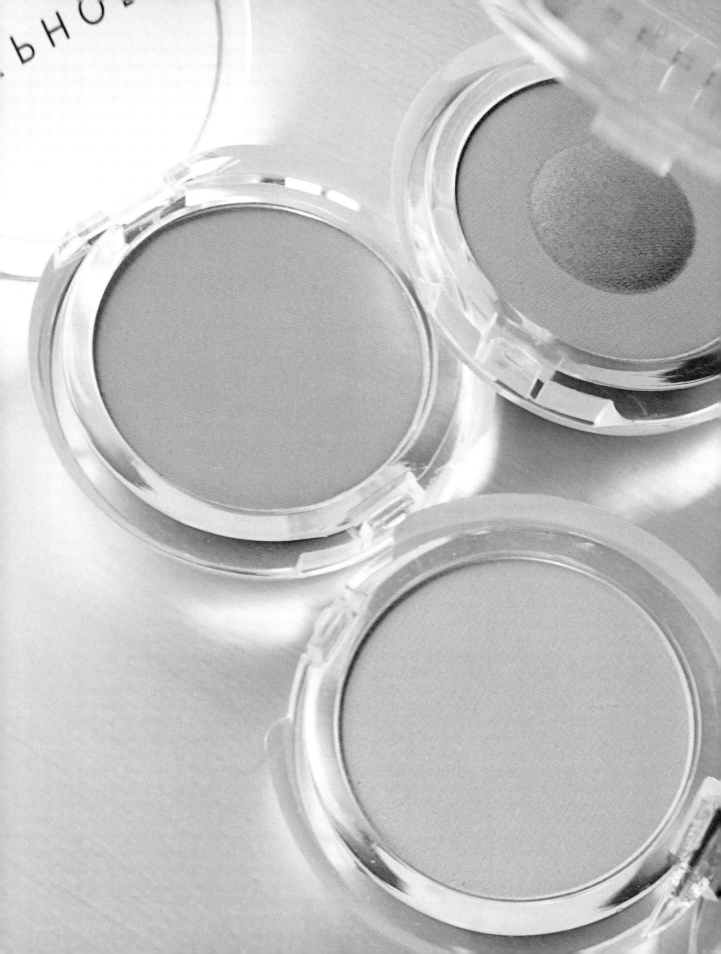

Eye shadow

- I like to play. Some days I want a sheer wash of color on my lids so I use Calvin Klein's Eye Color Wash. Most of the time I dust Paula Dorf's Aura powder shadow over my entire lid. It's almost skin-toned and evens out the eyelid color. I usually like a very natural eye for day, with any emphasis closer to the lash line.

Eyebrows

- Stila's brow powder has a great range of colors.

Blemishes

- Christian Dior makes a powder compact that will set your camouflage cream and cover anything. It's called Skin Compact. Just a dot on a Q-tip and your blemish is gone. If you like a little powder dusting at night, this does the job. Keep your powder at a minimum. We never want to look "powdered."

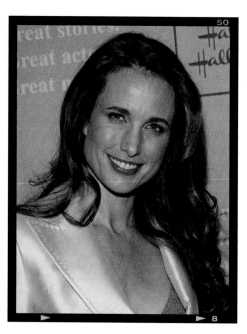

Andie McDowell has the look we want, natural and pretty without being obvious.

Lipstick and liner

- I use Lip Venom or City Lips to plump my lips and they really do.

- Always use a nude lip liner, on the light side, never on the dark side, unless you are using it to diminish your lip size. I have to admit I am a lipstick junkie. I buy tons, am never loyal to any one brand and change at a moment's notice. I simply love the hunt.

Shine

- I have tried everything: luminizers under, over, and mixed into my makeup and all different levels of shine. I am a sucker when they put them on my hand in the store. I love the way they twinkle, but I never love them on my face.

- Products that create shimmer and shine also enlarge pores, magnify puffiness, and draw attention to lines. It's not worth the trade-off.

GROWN-UP GIRL'S RULE FOR SHIMMER AND SHINE:
Use very, very sparingly, if at all.

Smothering Coverings

Cindy Crawford might be known for her beauty mark, but when you are a beauty like Cindy, you can make almost anything famous. The rest of us like to hide those little birthmarks, discolorations, moles, or curling iron burn marks. Who needs friends trying to dust the dirt off our faces or asking what happened to our cheek? The covering takes less time than the explanation.

Here's how to conceal problems:

- Apply your regular makeup, including the area to be covered.
- Start with an opaque cover-up like Joe Blasco's Amazing Concealer.
- Match the concealer to your skin tone.
- With a finger, pat the concealer on your hand. The heat from your hand will make it workable.
- Using your fingertip, apply to the area and slightly beyond.
- Blend out the edges *only*.
- If you need more coverage, apply and blend again.
- Apply powder to set the area. Use a clean powder puff. *Press* the powder into the skin, do not rub.
- Brush off the excess powder with a clean brush.
- Keep your hands and anyone else's hands off the area.

Spec Check

If you wear glasses do your final makeup check with them on. This is how others will see you. Glasses magnify. That eyeliner better be straight or everyone will know. Choose soft colors, use a light hand, and blend, blend, blend.

Makeup for eyeglass wearers:

- Apply your blush with your glasses on. Blush must start below the edge of your frame, so keep that in mind when choosing frames. No one looks good with amplified blush.
- Don't wear lash builder mascaras. Those tiny particles that build up your lashes look like gooey clumps behind glasses.

- Blend your foundation or tinted moisturizer around your eyes. Frames tend to collect makeup where they rest on the skin. This is not a collection to which we aspire.

- Every time you get a new prescription, put your glasses on to adjust your makeup. The stronger the glasses, the more subtle the application.

Sunshine and Candles

Pages and pages in women's magazines are dedicated to day and nighttime makeup. The difference is really very simple. Look at yourself in the light in which you will be seen.

For daytime, you must take your magnifying mirror to the brightest sunlight you can find. Also take your blending brush and sponge because you usually need to soften the edges. The bright light of day puts on view every start and stop of our makeup brushes. Soften all the edges of eye shadow, liner, and blush so you are hard pressed to tell where they begin and end. They should fade onto the face.

For nighttime, check your makeup under soft, dim lights. You will usually need a brighter, richer lipstick and a little more color on the cheeks. Take a stronger pink blush and dust only on the apples of the cheeks, on top of your regular daytime blush. This intensifies your color without looking fake. Make up your eyes as normal, adding a slightly thicker or darker line right at your lash line for more eye definition.

Never adjust your makeup under fluorescent lights in bathrooms and offices. Those old Clairol makeup mirrors that had daytime, nighttime, and fluorescent settings are off the market, as they should be.

MAKEUP MYTH: "YOU NEED MORE MAKEUP AT NIGHT."

You need a little more color in your makeup but not more amounts of makeup. Too much makeup cakes. Save the cake for dessert.

Grown-Up Girl's Makeup 101

- Keep your hands off your face. Hands harbor oil and bacteria that discolor your makeup and blemish the skin.

- Too little coverage is far better than too much.

- A lighter foundation is always safer than a darker one.

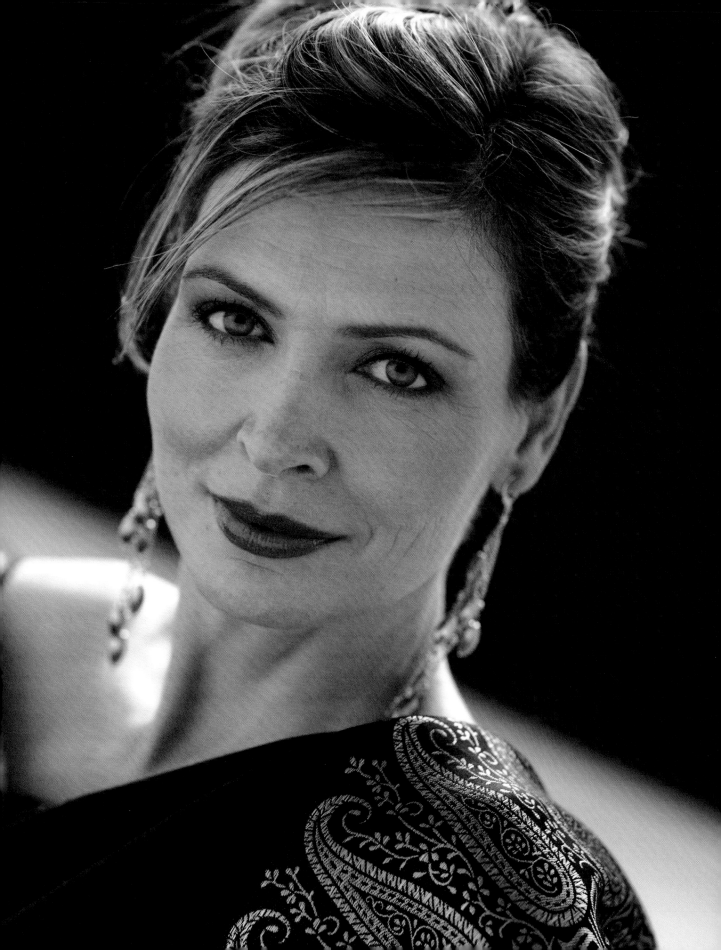

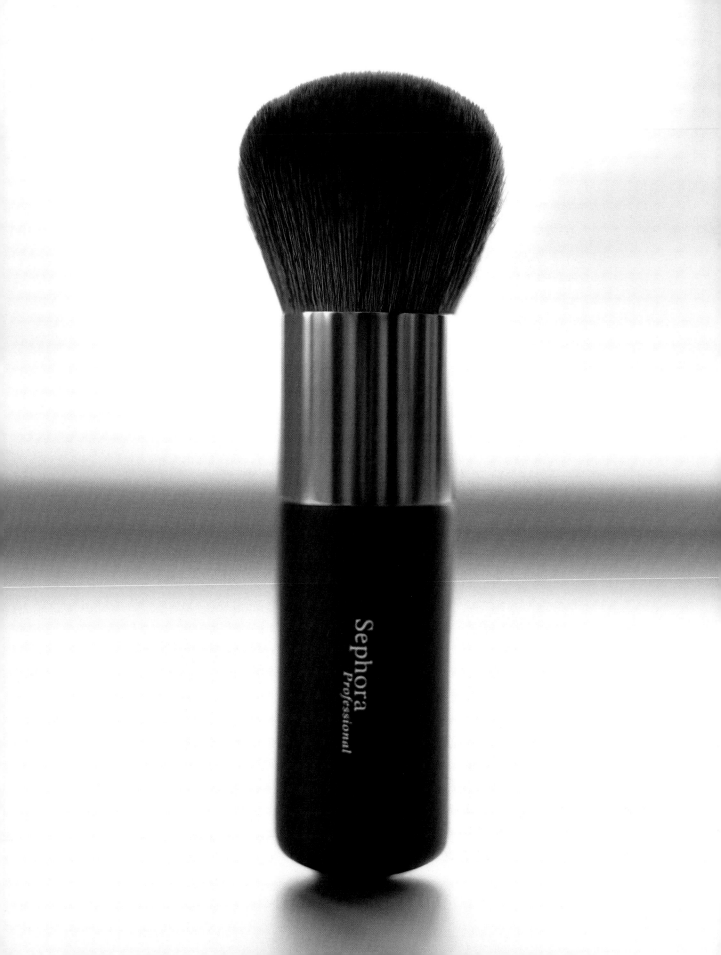

- Touch up makeup on the eyes and lips only. Accumulated oil and grime will make any added blush or foundation appear streaked and uneven.

- The stronger the color the less you use. Too much color overwhelms your features.

- Always check your compact mirror after eating for that dreaded spinach tooth. Sometimes even your best friends won't tell you. I wonder why?

- A nude lipliner pencil keeps lipgloss from bleeding past the lip line.

- Keep your makeup application to ten minutes or under. Complicated makeup will not give you that fresh, natural look. It will only look complicated.

- For puffy eyelids, apply a tiny dot of tan liquid foundation to the entire upper lid area. This is a very natural way of camouflaging puffiness.

- Refresh red, tired eyes with nonprescription, lightly tinted blue eye drops. They whiten the whites and make eyes look sparkling.

- If you're fading at night, line the inside rim of your lower eyes with a navy pencil.

The Freebies versus the Pros

Always keep current on makeup. That doesn't mean you have to constantly change, it simply means you might want to fine-tune. The more you learn about applying your own makeup, the more you will be able to pick and choose what really works for your face.

The free makeup applications at the department stores are really never free. The cosmetician needs to put the squeeze on you for products because she works on commissions and sales incentives. If she is pushing, pushing, pushing a plumping cream, think twice. That might be the item of the month and you might be her quota plump. Companies come out with new color campaigns each season. Don't get caught up in the hype. Go with what works for you. Take advantage of the so-called free sessions with the insight that you will buy a few items. Take what you like and incorporate it into your routine, disregard what you don't like. Remember there are no exacts in makeup.

Every few years visit a professional makeup artist at a salon. You will pay for the lesson and be nudged to buy products, but you will learn. In the end toss the bad and incorporate the good. No one knows your face like you do. If anyone starts shading your face, get up and grab your bag. Shading is for professional photo sessions only.

Robin Siegel is one of the best makeup artists in the business. For nine seasons she was the head makeup artist on *Friends*, and continues to work on the hottest shows. Her realistic approach is perfect for the grown-up girl. I was fortunate to have her do my makeup and I never looked better in a completely natural way.

Foundation:

Look for light to medium coverage, good ingredients, and easy application. Blend a couple of drops of foundation on your clean moisturized face to even out skin tones.

- M.A.C Select Tint SPF 15
- Armani
- Chanel, Chanel Crème Poudre
- Vitalumiere

Concealer:

Peachy colors neutralize blue undertones under the eyes. Yellow neutralizes redness.

- Clé de Peau
- Laura Mercier

Blush:

Cream blush well blended on the apples of the cheeks gives the look of a natural flush. Blush can brighten up your mood as well as your look.

- Stila Orchid convertible color
- M.A.C. Tickle Me Pink
- The best powder blushes are Cargo Cosmetics Catalina, Tonga, Molokai, and Mallorca: great packaging and easy-to-use beautiful color

Bronzer:

These give natural glow with easy application.

- Dr. Hauschka
- Chanel
- Clé de Peau

- Chanel, Clinique, Lancôme, or Clé de Peau in natural lip colors.
- Cargo or DuWop's Reverse Lip Liner is great to wear with lip gloss.

- Clé de Peau, M.A.C., Shiseido, and Chanel have great color and formula selections.

Experiment with different colors depending on the season and the outfit or find a signature color that helps define your personal style.

My favorite glosses are soft, not sticky.

- Clinique Glossimer, Lancôme, Chanel, M.A.C., or Shiseido
- For tinted lip balms try Clinique and M.A.C.

- M.A.C. Kohl pencil in Blooz (navy) or Prunella (deep plum) for lining inside the upper and lower lid is softer than black.
- M.A.C. Kohl pencil in Teddy is a beautiful shade of brown.
- Lancôme's Kohl Pencil in Black Coffee or Black Noir for more dramatic looks.

- M.A.C., Dr. Hauschka: always soften the line with eye shadow powder.

- Dr. Hauschka, Chanel, M.A.C. Pro Lash

Be aware of potential smudges under the eyes from mascara on the bottom lashes. Try applying mascara to bottom lashes first.

GROWN-UP GIRL'S FOUNDATION RULE:

If your foundation claims to cover everything it's the wrong one.

Only old-world movie stars still believe this. Work on making yourself flawless.

Our mothers covered their faces with makeup. We want to use makeup to brighten our faces, highlight our features, and enhance our texture. If you find you are using too much makeup to cover, find out the reason and correct it at the skin level. It must never look like you are wearing foundation. The purchasing switch starts in the forties. Before then the majority of your cosmetic money probably went for colors. After forty the greater part should go to treatment products.

GROWN-UP GIRL'S MAKEUP RULE:

We don't need less makeup as we get older, we just need it to look like less.

The reality is you need about the same amount of makeup with a lighter application. As we age our coloring fades. That definition we had at twenty softens into one overall tone with each decade. Makeup gives us back our definition. The love affair continues.

Diet Brows

When it comes to eyebrows, skinny is out, fat is in.

Unfortunately eating French fries and Baskin Robbin's Chocolate Chocolate Chunk ice cream has nothing to do with increasing the size of your brows. Years of waxing and tweezing do. A thin, forties- or fifties-style brow flatters Kate Moss. If you were born in the forties, fifties, or sixties, that's probably not the case for you.

So how do you get a thicker brow? You let it grow. Now I know you are saying, "My brows won't grow. I've tried and what grows are unwanted strays." I promise you that those unwanted strays will thicken and soften your brow line if you have patience. The average eyebrow follicle takes anywhere from fifty-five to sixty-five days to grow after it is plucked.

Don't pull anything right under your brow or anything right next to the brows between your eyes. Some hairs will grow in sticking straight out but they will fall in place once they are long enough. Some will seem like they are too far away from your brow line but a dab of brow color will fill in the holes until another one comes along.

Once one row fills in, start the next until you have the desired thickness. It may take a year, but they will grow. Have them professionally shaped once you have some growth. Tell the cosmetician that you are letting them grow in and to please not remove

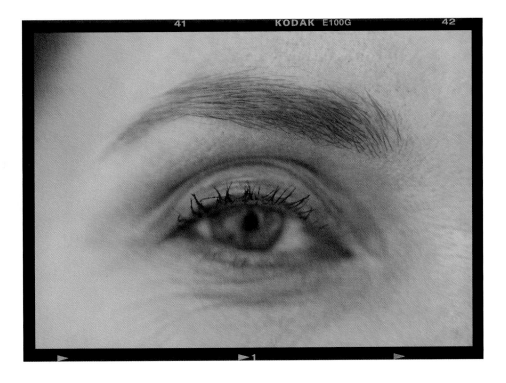

any thickness. If she gets out the wax, get up and run. Waxing is good for bushy brows, but it is *never* good for shaping brows. That can *only* be done with tweezers, taking one hair at a time. It is impossible to control wax the way you can control tweezers. Cosmeticians love wax because it takes one-fifth of the time of tweezing. You are not concerned with saving their time, you are interested in saving your brows.

Look at pictures of yourself when you were in your teens, before you discovered tweezers. That shape is your natural shape and one you should try to achieve, only with a neat, well-groomed appearance.

Brow Paint

If you color, color, color as I recommend, you might need to include your eyebrows. Lovely chestnut hair with gray eyebrows is like a designer knockoff bag that has a Target logo showing. They give away your secrets. Brows don't have to match your hair, but they do have to blend with it. Some pencils or brow powders will do the trick. If not, you need to tint. Your hair colorist can do this for you but you will need the formula for a touch-up at home. Brows fade and grow much faster than hair color.

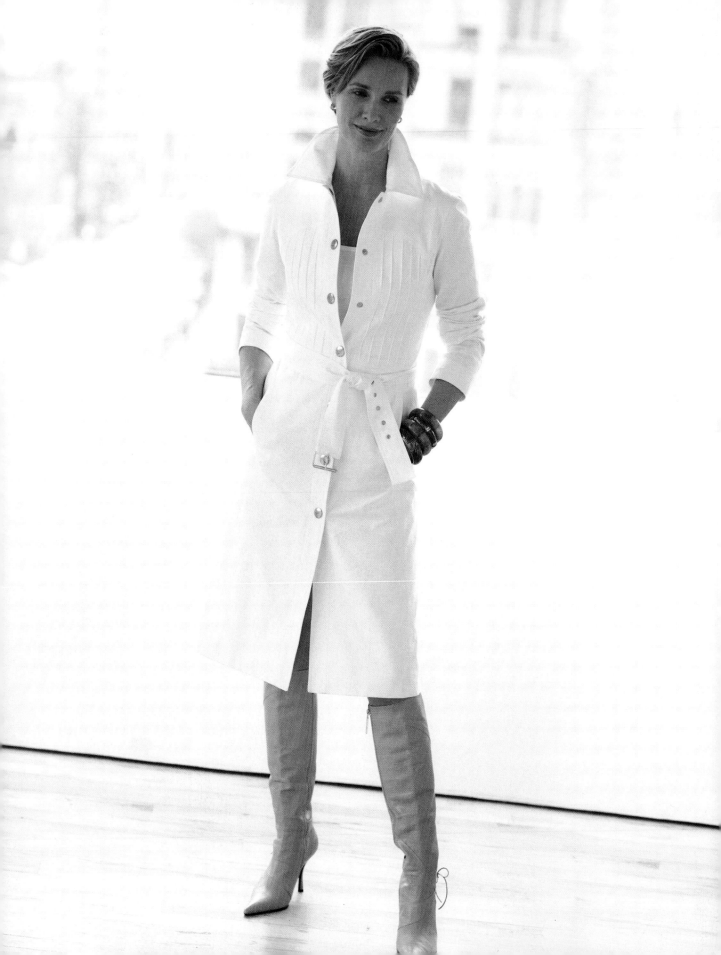

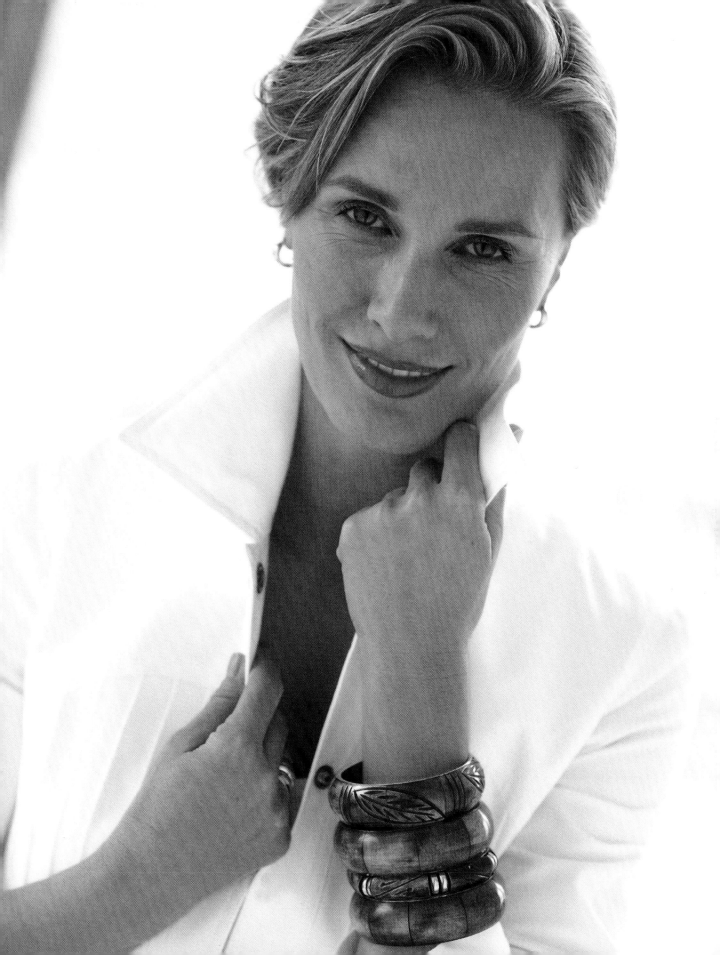

- Adjust your home hair color slightly lighter for brows.

- Blondes should be a dark blonde to light brown.

- Redheads could try a nutmeg brown.

- Brunettes can match their brows to their hair.

- Leave color on in ten-minute increments, check color. Maximum time is thirty minutes.

- If your brow shape is not well defined, use a brow stencil to help you define the shape (available from M.A.C., Anastasia Brows, or Fran Wilson Instant Brow Stencils).

Mascara Surrogate

Do you dream of retiring your mascara wand or of having semipermanent dark, smoldering eyelashes? Products to tint your lashes sound good: wake up in the morning with eyelashes, swim without makeup. But the reality is that tinting doesn't take the place of mascara because there is absolutely no thickening. Yes, you do look better in the morning but the tint fades more quickly than anyone will admit.

Think of how the chlorine from a pool bleaches your hair and skin. Those delicate little tinted lashes will bleach out in one or two splashes. Save your money. It's a good concept that does not translate to reality.

To Tattoo or Not to Tattoo

Did you ever think about a tattoo at this age? Don't cross it off your list. If you have waxed your eyebrows to oblivion, have ultrasensitive eyes that tear off most makeup, or a lip line that seems to be diminishing you might want to consider tattooing, or as it has been renamed for cosmetic purposes, *permanent makeup.*

The stipulation is, that unlike the younger generation, you want all your tattoos to look completely natural. Don't decide that Goldie Hawn lips would look good on you, they won't. Here are a few tips:

Eyebrows should blend, not match, with your hair color and follow your eye shape. Go to a professional makeup artist first, have them pencil in the correct shape and color. Don't leave it up to the person tattooing to decide what brow shape suits you. On that note, make sure your tattoo artist is a skilled technician. Tattooed eyeliner should be a medium or dark brown; black is too harsh. Less and lighter is always better.

Follow the natural shape of your eye as if you were filling in between your eyelashes with pencil. If you line the lower lashes, make it one or two shades lighter than the top liner. This will keep your eyes looking open and fresh. All liner should consist of small dots, nothing should resemble a solid line.

Tattooed lipliner should be a nude, natural color, matching your lips. You don't want it to look like you have on heavy lip pencil. Understated is what you want, not extreme.

GROWN-UP GIRL'S TATTOO RULE:

Never do anything trendy with anything permanent.

The tattoo in this case is a definite "not." Who wants more emphasis put on their upper arms?

BEAUTY MYTH: "ONLY BAD GIRLS HAVE TATTOOS."

Today good girls, bad girls, and girls needing a permanent fix have tattoos. Tattooing is not meant to totally replace makeup, it's to enhance it.

The Scent of a Woman

Fragrance precedes us as we walk in a room. It defines us as we kiss hello or hug good-bye. Some women are associated with a particular scent; others change fragrances as they change outfits. It is important for maintenance purposes that your scent not be overwhelming or too sweet. These scream "dated." Think of the elevator you step into that reeks of perfume. We never, ever want to reek. If you get compliments on your perfume from a distance they are not compliments, they are warnings.

In high school I was a "Shalimar girl." My boyfriend bought me my first bottle of Shalimar because his old girlfriend wore it. I still dated him, but hey, I was only sixteen. Years passed and I was in the department store doing my ritual perfume search. There sat the Shalimar bottle. I was once again sixteen, for about thirty minutes. The lovely Shalimar turned sickly sweet.

Our body chemistry changes as we grow. The only way you can tell what a fragrance will smell like on you is to wear it for an extended period of time. Those little paper sticks they spray with perfume in the stores are good to let you sniff and get an idea if this is something you might like to try. Don't ever buy a fragrance based on a paper stick.

Spray it and wear it first. Smell it in an hour, smell it in two hours, smell it in six hours. Does it last, do you love it? Don't waste your money on something that smelled wonderful on a friend until you try it on yourself.

You can have several fragrances: a light one for day and a richer one for evening. You can have your bedroom scent that never sees the light of day. Scents are signature items. Our signature should be a positive, memorable statement.

FRAGRANCE MYTH: "YOU CAN TELL A WOMAN BY HER SCENT."

What can you tell? A good scent should accompany a woman, not announce her.

The Grown-Up Girl's Beauty Maintenance Goal

Beauty may indeed be in the eyes of the beholder, but it's also the way we see ourselves. See yourself as ageless. Adapt your makeup as you evolve as a woman. Don't lock into what you did, instead, improve each year with what you are doing. Experiment with new colors, new techniques, and new scents. Don't stand still. Look at the abundance of beauty magazines. They are testimony to the ever-changing field of beauty. We are testimony to the ever-changing woman. Take what works for you and add it in your mix. You must be an adventurous beauty to be an ageless one.

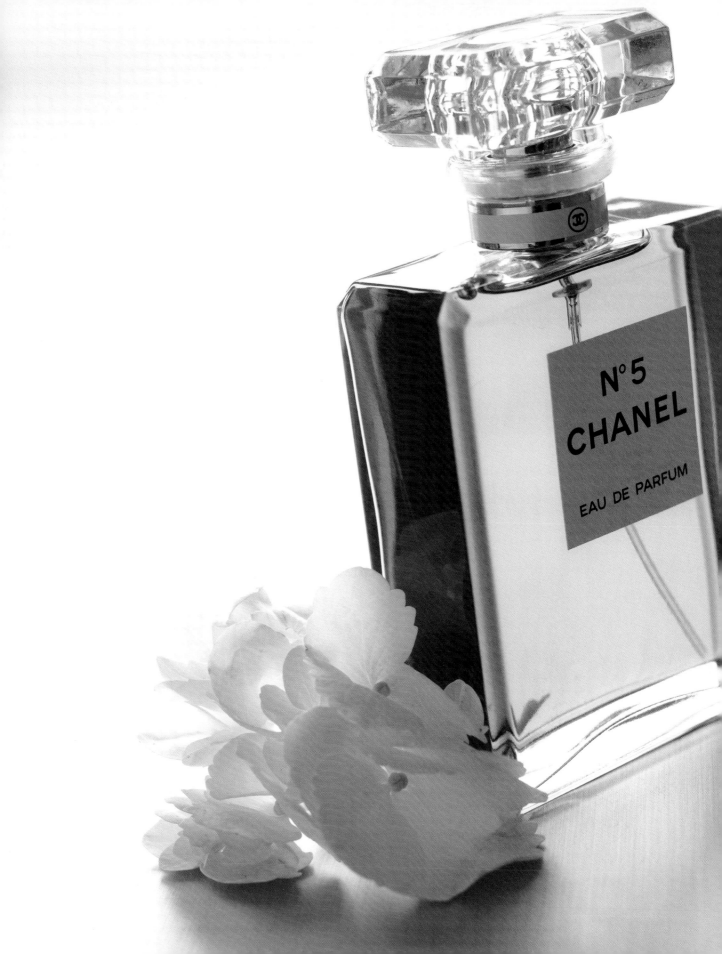

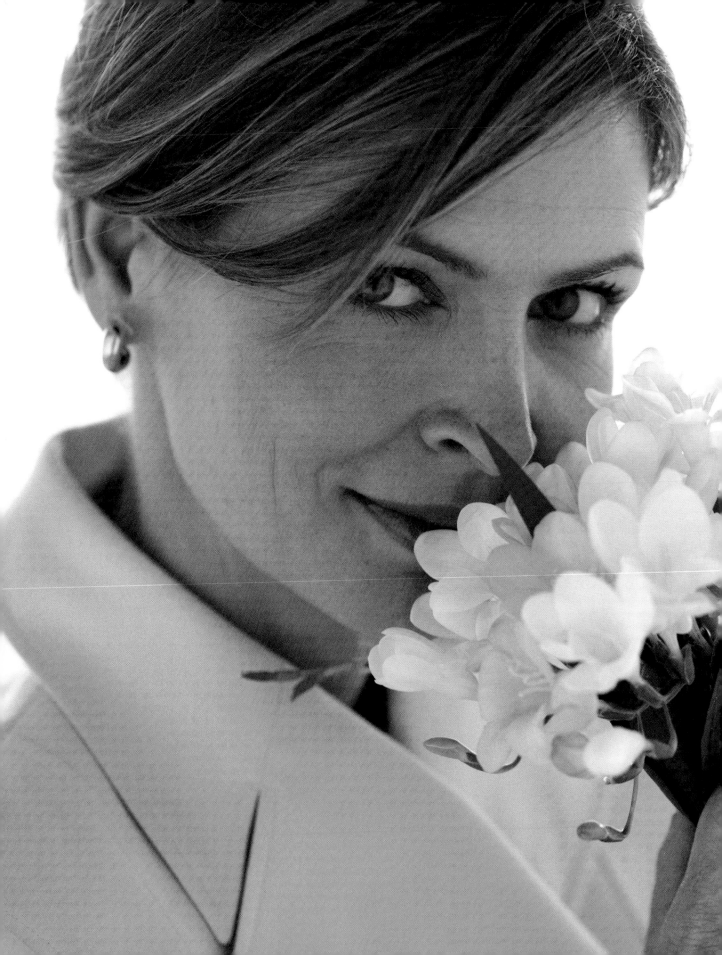

PART THREE

And More...

Maintenance doesn't stop with fashion and beauty. Our attitude, health, lifestyle, and family and friends also require maintenance. We are not just about appearance, we are about being a complete person. We only reach our objectives when we have all the elements, the inner with the outer, in place. The myth "all beauty comes from within" is half of the equation. If we don't have inner beauty, we can't be beautiful human beings. It's the balance between the two. I feel inner beauty all begins with attitude.

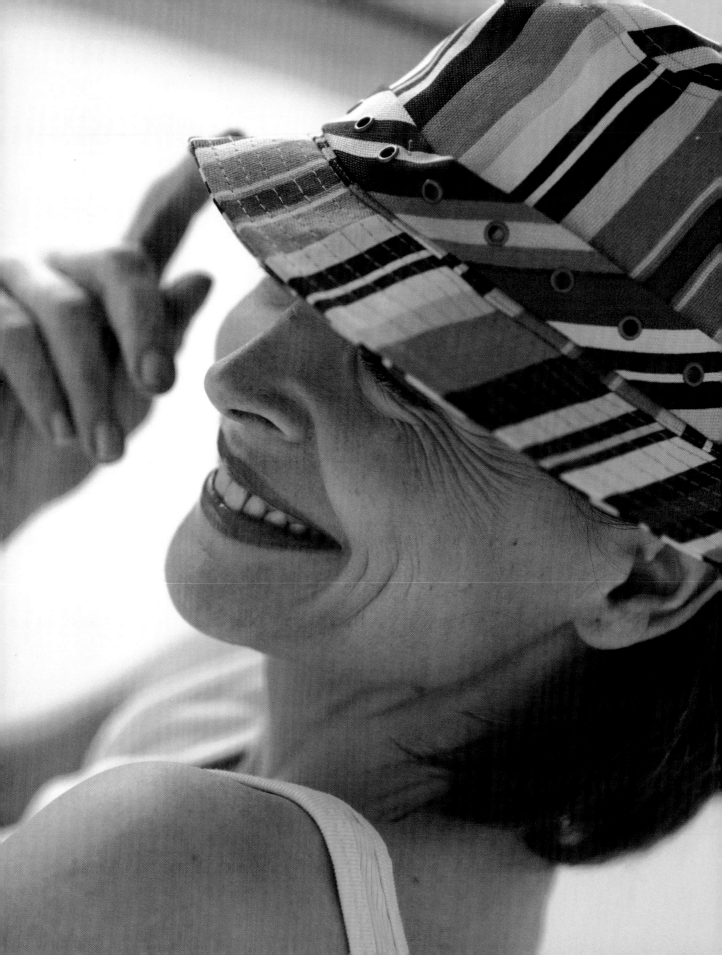

the Mind

Attitude

One evening a few years ago, I joined my husband and another couple for a business dinner. These can be tough because the men get right down to business and usually I am left with a woman I have never met. Sometimes it's a delightful evening and sometimes it's not.

This one was all work. Across from me sat a beautiful woman filled with negativity and anger and I was her sounding board for the night. Two and a half hours later as we drove home I said to my husband, "Don't ever expose me to that woman again." A negative attitude ages a woman right before your very eyes. A positive attitude makes a woman more attractive.

No matter how much we maintain our bodies, if we don't maintain our attitudes as well we will never be the complete women we are capable of being. We must work to be positive. Life and its experiences can often make us disillusioned. We must turn it around. We must make the roller-coaster ride of life a high, not get stuck in the lows. We must make the journey our reward.

Can you change your attitude? I believe you can.

Fashionably Minded

As a culture we are way too obsessed with age. It doesn't help that the media puts a number on every woman and a spin on the importance of the lower numbers. No wonder so many women lie about their age. I have to ask myself why the focus on youth? I find people far more interesting, gracious, and charming as they age. I find women more beautiful and, as singer/songwriter John Mellencamp put it so well, "Men aren't worth a damn until they are forty." Do I believe this because I am of that unfashionable age? Perhaps. The number is not important, the person is.

Today we really are ageless. You can look ageless if you so desire, but that's not the final objective. Ageless is as much about the state of mind as it is about the state of body. Happiness begins in the mind. It's not about what we have, who we are, or what we look like. It's about us. Are we born happy? I doubt it. Can we attain happiness? I believe we can, but we have to want it and work at it. Waking up in the morning happy and sustaining it throughout the day takes hard work, but then, doesn't anything worth having?

You have probably heard the saying, "The lines you have at fifty are the lines you deserve." I feel it holds many truths. The women who smile a lot have upturned smile lines. The ones who frown have downturned ones.

GROWN-UP GIRL'S AGE RULE:

Forget about it!

The Start of Something New

Keep fresh.

Be open to the new. If you give up on your looks you will look defeated.

If you give up on your mind you will be boring and bored.

If you don't care, no one else will.

But you do care, we all do, so continue to keep your mind open, shake up your patterns, forget your chronological age, and live your desired age.

It all starts with something new: something for yourself that expands your horizons, makes you stretch without exercising, and takes you out of your comfort realm. Anne Abernathy is the oldest woman ever to compete in the Winter Olympics. At the age of fifty-one she has competed in six Olympics. Julie Andrews at sixty-nine is busier than she has ever been with writing, acting, and directing.

I have several friends who at the ages of forty and fifty went back to college. They completely changed their careers. Age never factored into their decisions to make the changes. Why should it? We are never too old to learn and change—unless we think we are.

GROWN-UP GIRL'S BOREDOM RULE:

If you are bored with life you will be boring.

It's hard to learn at any age, but it's always rewarding.

Delete Your Spam

Our heads are filled with junk mail. We run on overload most of the time. We worry about things we can't control. It's time to press the delete button. If worries keep you awake at night, practice replacing them with positive thoughts. For every pessimistic notion that enters your head, think of an optimistic solution.

Negativity drags us and everyone around us down. It takes up time and energy that should be used for positive action and thoughts. It's unrealistic to eliminate all the negativity in your life, but you can start to control it. Does the news depress you? Cut back on your viewing. Do parts of the daily newspapers put you in a funk? Skip those sections. Is a friend or family member wearing you out with their lack of enthusiasm for life? Restrict their time allotment in your life. Find solutions to cynical influences. Don't complain about them—solve them.

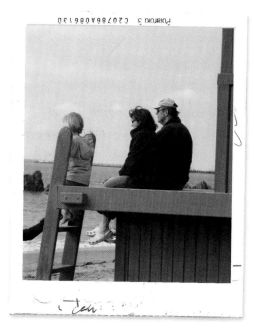

Pick a calming place to fill your head with optimistic thoughts.

LIFESTYLE MYTH: "YOU CAN TURN A NEGATIVE PERSON AROUND."

I don't think so; in fact, they will most likely try to turn you around. Negativity loves company—don't be theirs.

Brain Exercises

Keep those brain waves in constant motion. Expand your knowledge of something that interests you. Explore all the things you wish you knew how to do. "It's too late" or "I can't find the time" are weak excuses. Why is it we continuously find the time when we have to? It's always the right time to grow and learn. Exercise keeps your body young. Continue that exercise in your brain. Enroll in an extension class. Join or form a book club, volunteer in a worthwhile organization, start a new career, go back to school for a degree. Anything and everything is possible if you just try.

GROWN-UP GIRL'S LEARNING RULE:
We are never too old unless we think we are.

Maybe some do, but we still have plenty left. Current research says if you keep your mind active and stimulated you can actually gain intelligence.

Small Packages

Some of my favorite attitude adjusters come in small packages. The balance of life, love, and total acceptance with young children and animals cannot be compared. They need you and they love you unconditionally. Can anyone resist that kind of worship?

It's hard to be in a bad mood when a three-year-old greets you running with outstretched arms or a puppy is gently licking your cheek. A playful kitten dancing at your feet can make you smile after a difficult day. My father never wanted to live anywhere that had the name "retirement" associated with it. He chose to live in a community with young children and lots of dogs. "Who wants to be surrounded by people who are all my age?" was his rationale. Watching him interact with small children and the neighbor's golden lab made me realize he was absolutely right.

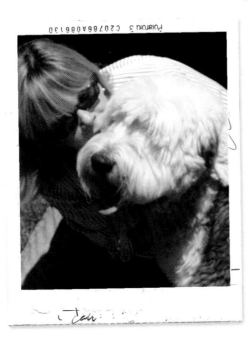

This is Nigel, our Old English sheepdog. We like to think of him as a person in a dog suit.

Trash Talk

Just recently I was at a luncheon table of over-forty women when a young, beautiful twenty-something stopped by to talk. All eyes looked her up and down. She had youth. Every woman at the table was trying to look younger, but nothing takes the place of natural youth and it was apparent on the faces of several of the women. You can pick out who is happy with the way she looks and who isn't.

Jealousy is not a pretty thing. It reveals itself on your face. Envy is not to be envied. Everyone around you can sense it and you don't look good. Don't be angry that someone is younger or more beautiful than you, don't be jealous or envious. Enjoy their youth and beauty. Contentment looks extremely attractive.

When the young woman moved on to another table some returned to their luncheon chatter, while others tore her apart. Her dress was too this, her figure too that. "Why would anyone wear that putrid color?" "That is a knockoff if I ever saw one." Picky, picky, picky. Youth might indeed be wasted on the young but age brings confidence, experience, and hopefully wisdom. Focus on your assets, not someone else's. Watch someone's face as they talk trash. It's not what we want our faces to look like.

The Cynical Staircase

Cynical thinking leads to a downward spiral. Yes, many things are changing, and we must accept the changes and modify the ones we can for the better. Don't focus on the downbeat. Every year produces more information than we can store. Are we overdue for a spring cleaning? So you forget things. Don't attribute it to a "senior moment." We need to eliminate "PMS Syndrome," "The Mature Moment," "Menopause Memory," or any other cutesy media-coined phrase that put us into a negative category.

Think back, how many times have you opened the refrigerator, forgetting what you were looking for . . . in your teens and twenties? At some point, everyone forgets why they walked into a room. It is only as we grow up that we tend to focus on it and blame it on age. Blame it on forgetting and then forget it.

Forget the cliché "the good old days." Live in the good days right now. Embrace progress. Welcome change. Pessimism is aging. Be open, be cheeky, be contemporary, and you will be forever young. Progress is for *all* of us. Take advantage!

My Way

Frank Sinatra might have made it his theme song, but it shouldn't be ours. Yes, it's true, as we get older we do know the best ways to do things—or at least we think we do. Keep your "my ways" to yourself.

Respect the people in your life and give them the benefit of the doubt. Believe me, they will ask if they need your help. If they don't, let that be okay, too.

Why is it necessary to correct a mate over a small detail like time or place when they are in the midst of telling a story to other couples over a lovely dinner? Who really cares about the time or the place? Correcting doesn't make the mate look wrong, it makes the person doing the correcting look controlling. Let it go. Don't put your values on those you love. Love their values just like you did when you first fell in love.

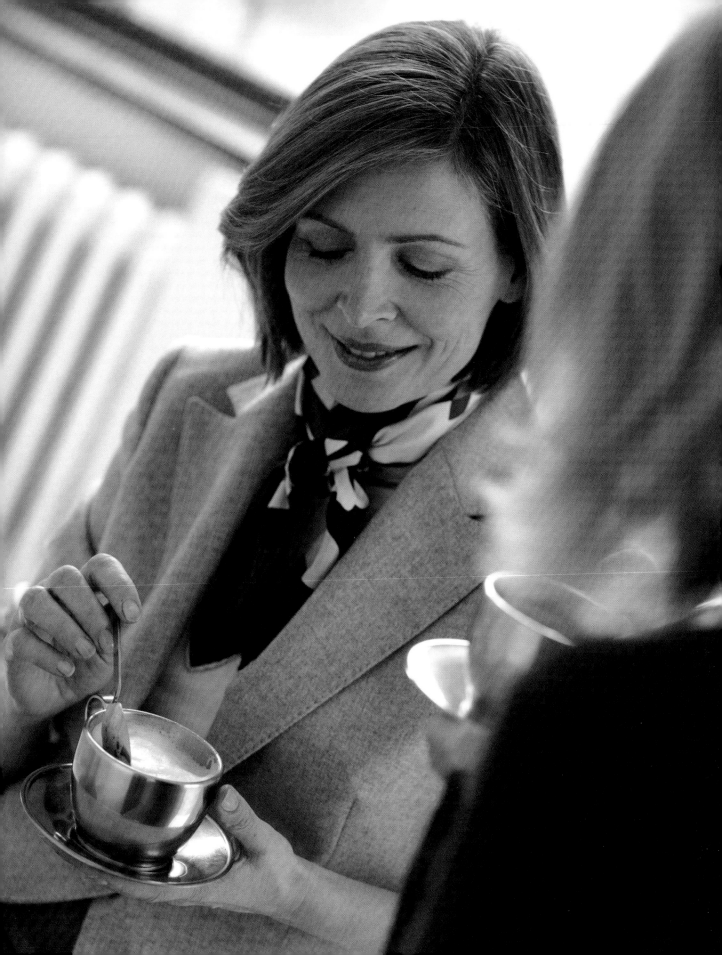

CHAPTER NINE

Friends and Family

Family and friends are the foundation of life. When you have a supportive family and wonderful friends you are indeed a rich person. Accepting family and selecting friends has been a big learning experience for me.

Expectations

I have always been a person with extremely high expectations. It's a good thing because it motivates me, but on the downside, I am easily disappointed.

I love the holidays and celebrations. Rallying a family of four grown kids, three of my husband's and one of mine, is not always easy, and they are all great kids. When we try to get together someone is almost always missing. They have their own lives, other families, and obligations. So the perfect holidays don't always turn out the way I envisioned. My importance is not their importance. Intellectually I can understand it, but emotionally I have a hard time dealing with it. I want everyone to be around, and everyone to have a good time. Instead of concentrating on who did come, I concentrate on who didn't make it. Instead of concentrating on who's having fun, I worry about who isn't happy. I feel because I have set the tone for family traditions that our family will follow in my footsteps. I am learning that they are busy making their own footsteps.

Fear Fences

I have one older relative who drives the freeways and the highways on a daily basis. I have another who fears them. I have one friend who gets on an airplane the way others get into a car. I have another who fears them. Why do women put perimeters on life as they grow up? Does experience and knowledge make us fearful? Does it make us limit our lives at a time when we should be broadening them?

Fear builds fences around life. Fear of failing can make you stop taking chances and eliminate the possibility of success. Fear of intimacy might make you pass up a friendship or love of a lifetime. Fear of commitment keeps relationships on the surface. Fear of getting better might keep others from expecting more of you.

We need to change "I'm afraid" to "I'm willing to try." Only if we try will we experience all that life can be. The possibilities are limitless if we take down our fences.

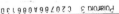

The Multisandwich Family

I'm not talking a club sandwich on wheat toast. I'm talking about managing the responsibilities of aging parents and children at the same time. The pressures come from all directions. We are all living longer and with that come more responsibilities.

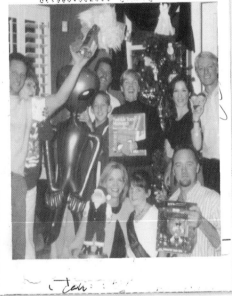

The hardest lesson I have had to learn is to let parents be independent. They want and need to make their own decisions and even if we don't always agree, we do owe them the respect of letting them make those decisions. My father didn't want to go on kidney dialysis. He knew it meant the end of his life. I didn't understand it or agree with it but he deserved the dignity to make his own choice. It is very difficult to watch a loved one go down a path you feel is wrong. I have now learned through trial, error, and lots of trying to control, that it is important to allow them to go down their own paths.

This is my multisandwich family at our annual holiday gathering. Who wouldn't laugh if you received a blow up alien or a rock 'n' roll Santa for a gift?

We all want to protect our children from the mistakes we made. We want them to be perfect, just as we wish we were. But we're not and neither are they. Accepting them for who they are is the kindest gift we can give them.

There's truth to the saying "the most supportive thing you can do for your children is to allow them to fail." It sounds harsh but now I would have to say I agree, having tried to save both my parents and my children many times when I should have just let them be.

Inheritance versus Selection

We inherit our families. Sometimes that's a good thing and sometimes it isn't. Is there a certain obligation to family? Must we be there no matter what? Is blood really thicker than water? I believe just because someone is related to you doesn't mean you have to like them. People have to earn the love and respect of their family just as they do with friends. Sure, we cut family more slack, but where do we draw the line? We have all seen a destructive relative devastate a family. How can that be okay? We've seen families abuse each other. Is that all right? If you have toxic next of kin, buffer yourself. Rise above the situation. Accept the fact that you can't change *them,* but *you* can change. Do what you need to do to protect yourself. Create some distance, enough to keep you healthy. Is this painful? Absolutely. But you will probably find out that the relationship you lost sleep over was not as good as you thought it was. If you don't take care of yourself, who will?

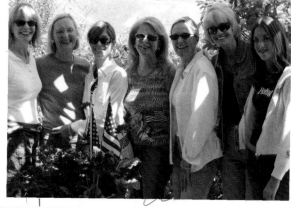

Family and friends at a Fourth of July gathering. Your inheritances and acquisitions should make you smile.

With friends we have more room to negotiate. So then why do we let toxic friends into our lives and keep them there? Why do we become the breeding ground for their negativity? Stop! Edit your friends. It might be a little difficult in the beginning but you will feel so much better in the long term.

I had to make a deletion in my life. My once vibrant friend became overwhelmed with life's disappointments. Lunches and dinners with her were filled with talk of how bad things were. When I tried to turn it around she only became resentful. She was exhausting.

Finally, I knew I had to move on after hours on the phone hearing her negativity. I am sure she feels I am insensitive to her needs. I am sure she feels abandoned, but I feel abandoned as well. I lost the friend I once had, I can't get her back, and yet I can't be with who she has become. I believe in taking responsibility for your life. I believe you can change things for the better. Our contrasting viewpoints are no longer compatible for either of us. Do I miss her? I miss who she used to be.

Friendship should be a good thing. Friends ought to nurture you, and make you laugh, share, and grow. Would you keep a pair of shoes in your closet that hurt your feet every time you wore them? Would you continue to wear them even though they gave you blisters? Don't let friends hurt or blister you. That's not a friend, that's a foe. The saying "misery loves company" is not a myth, it's a reality.

Green-Eyed Friends

In my late twenties my life took a giant leap forward. I moved from a modest house in Los Angeles to a beautiful house in the upscale area of Palos Verdes. Friends came by the first week to see my new home. It turned out to be a very interesting, insightful, and eye-opening experience. You could tell the green-eyed friends the minute they saw the house. It put a damper on the sharing, and a sour note on some of the relationships.

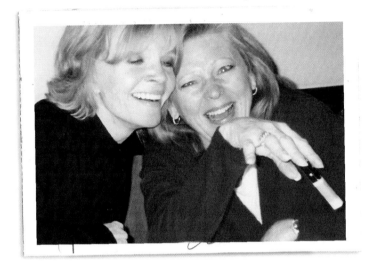

How long has it been since you laughed so hard you cried? When my friend superglued her finger to the glue tube, we fell apart. What a perfect fit: friendship and laughter!

I have known my best friend since junior high. We are still great friends even though our lives took very different turns. She loves to travel, whereas I love to be home. When she came to look at my Palos Verdes purchase she was ecstatically happy for me. When I first appeared on television she was my biggest fan. When I landed a magazine column she told all her friends to buy the magazine. When I sold my first book she bought more copies than anyone. When she had her son she asked me to be his godmother. We have both reached our goals in different ways. There is no room for any green eyes in our friendship.

FRIENDSHIP MYTH: "FRIENDS ARE ALWAYS HAPPY FOR YOU."

Your true friends are sincerely happy for you. The others are really only associates.

Youngsters

A funny thing happens to single women as they pass forty. The selection of good men narrows drastically. It seems that the majority of men over forty want much younger women, and the inequity is they can usually get them. Unlike women, they don't have to necessarily be in good shape, be stylish, or fascinating. Walking, breathing, working men are in demand.

I guess most men aren't interested in conversation or stimulation anywhere above their waist or there wouldn't be so many terrific single grown-up girls. But the tides are changing, the tables are turning. Many women over forty find older men stuck in their ways.

The solution? Turn to younger men. Madonna found it with an Englishman. Susan Sarandon proved it long ago with Tim Robbins, and now Demi Moore has splashed it on the covers of major magazines with Ashton Kutcher. Ageless women need ageless men. The chronological years are not the issue when it comes to relationships. Thirty, forty, fifty, or sixty, it's about the person, not the numbers. When friends want to play matchmaker, stop asking how old he is and start asking who he is. If we want to be ageless women we need to be open to ageless men.

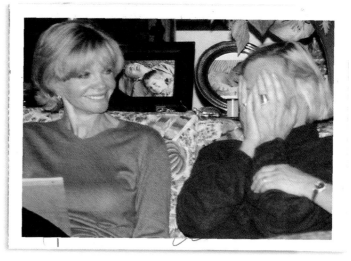

We are never, ever, too mature to giggle.

SINGLE GROWN-UP GIRL'S RULE FOR MEN:

Choose the man not the number.

In Your Own Backyard

Is that perfect mate eluding you? Have you decided all the good ones are gone? Are you discouraged, disinterested, and destined to be forever single? Perhaps not. Possibly he is already a part of your life. Maybe he is that special person you always love to talk with, who understands, makes you laugh, and is easy to be around. Take a look at the one you consider "just a friend."

At a Fourth of July gathering, my single sister was intrigued by two happily married couples having a conversation about how friends turned into lovers. She kept asking questions, and finally 'fessed up that she had been thinking about one of her best friends lately and wondering what might have been. Hearing their stories she realized that it still could happen. We all encouraged her to put the idea out there to this friend and explore the possibilities. We even made plane reservations for her to go for a visit.

She made the phone call but canceled her reservations because he immediately hopped on a plane to come to her. It seems he had the same thought. The adjustment from friend to lover didn't take long. The foundation for a relationship had been there all along. Now she has moved lock, stock, and barrel to be with him. Friends as lovers? It's certainly worth consideration. Take another look around you. That perfect mate might be right in your own backyard.

Just a Face-Lift and Hairstyle Away

How honest can we be with our friends? One of my closest friends is an amazing lady. She is smart, compassionate, and loving. We are as different as night and day when it comes to maintenance. She is a naturalist who maintains her weight with any outdoor activity. Her life is filled with family, friends, travel, and work. The only time you hear the tiniest bit of a complaint coming from her is when she says "Life would be perfect if I had someone to share it with." She so deserves someone. The reason she doesn't have anyone? Sorry guys, but most grown-up men are shallow. They are into looks and young grown-up girls.

She never asks me for any appearance advice. I think she feels I am in another orbit. Yet I wish she would. I often long to offer suggestions but I'm not willing to risk her friendship. You see, in my fashionista mind she is just a face-lift and a good hairstyle away from finding that mate. The outdoorsy lifestyle has taken a natural toll on her face. She has pretty features that simply need a little tweaking. Her hair is short and natural and easy to maintain. It fits into her life but not into what's flattering. I know firsthand she is not opposed to plastic surgery, so why doesn't she want to make the changes? She might feel someone needs to love her for who she is and they will— once they get past their shallow maleness. She's just not playing the game the way it's played today. She doesn't have a level playing field. She is competing with women who do. Will she ever find her perfect mate? If only I could tell her she's just a hairstyle and face-lift away. Perhaps now I have.

The beauty myth that you only get a face-lift for yourself is not entirely true. Sometimes maintenance is the means to your goals. Is that shallow? Perhaps.

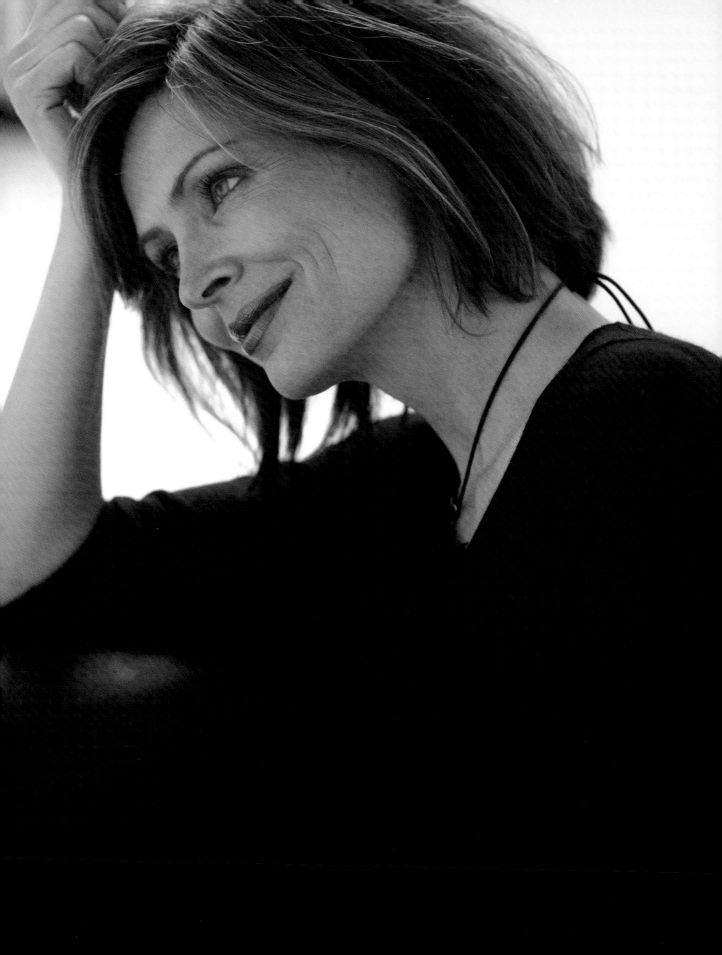

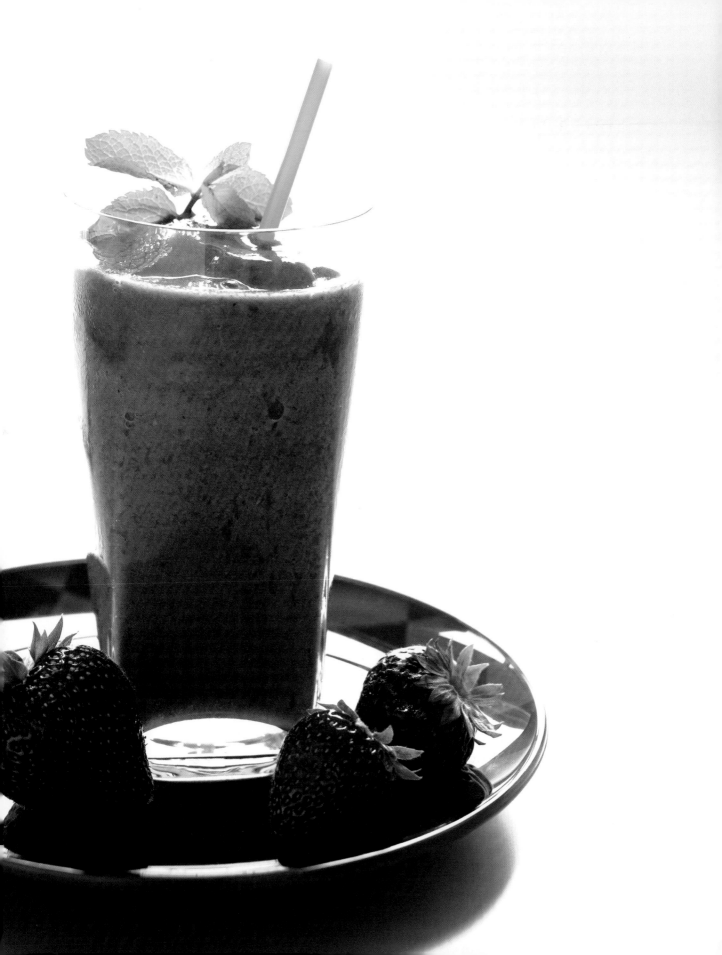

CHAPTER TEN

Fit Food

Dieting is an American pastime. You just mention the word and the buzz starts. "Have you read . . . ?" "Have you tried . . . ?" "Fifteen pounds in ten days." We are diet-crazed, diet-obsessed, and on diet overload. Personally I think we should delete the word. Diets imply success. I just don't feel they deliver.

Forty-and-Counting Bodies

What happens to the body after forty? You might already know because it's happening to yours. If not, let me break it to you gently. I call it the two S's. It slows and it spreads.

It doesn't happen overnight and it may not hit until you are well into your fifties, but it hits. All of a sudden you notice a thickening around your waist, a little dimple effect on your thighs and buttocks that's not associated with adorable, and what seems to be little pouches of extra skin. Where did it come from? You're doing everything the same but your body is not.

It's all about maintenance. Changing your eating habits and exercising is the *only* long-term way to keep your weight under control. You must eat healthy to be healthy. You have to eat less to weigh less. It's essential to move around to stay fit.

You have to retrain your brain. There is no simple answer. There is no magical diet. Yes, celebrities promote a diet that keeps them slim and the photographs in their books support their theory. But how many of them have personal trainers, special food prepared daily, and surgical procedures to carve and trim their bodies?

GROWN-UP GIRL'S DIET RULE:

Don't dwell on diets. Dwell on eating healthy.

DIET MYTH: "DIET YOUR WAY TO HEALTH."

Please change that to *eat* your way to health.

Eating Adjustments for Slowing Metabolism

Why, when I do the same exercise routine that had kept my weight down for years, does it no longer work? Because I am not the same and neither are you. Our metabolism slows down, even if our lives don't.

How can we gear it up? By changing our routines. The types of food you eat and the way you prepare them should not be the same at forty and fifty as they were at twenty.

THE LATEST DIET

My philosophy and the philosophy of everyone I know that stays in shape is to move more and eat less. A diet for a couch potato can't work. It's the simple mathematics of calories in, calories burned.

Yes, diets can trick your body to burn more fat and to drop pounds quickly. But they can't trick your body to be forever slim. Only you can do that with the combination of eating better, eating less, and exercising more.

HABIT MYTH: "HABITS ARE HARD TO BREAK."

No, they are actually pretty easy to break—it's just hard to maintain those breaks.

NOONERS

Change your eating patterns. Eat your biggest meal at noontime. You need more energy during the day and you have more time to burn off the calories. All those lady-like lunchtime salads should be your dinnertime salads. Making the switch will allow you to eat a bit more of what you love. Keep your dinners light and early. I have friends that think you are only chic if you dine at 8 P.M. Well, I can't be that chic. My metabolism won't let me.

SCALED DOWN DISHES

While visiting one very slim and fit friend for an overnight visit we decided to make a bowl of cereal with fresh fruit for our "diet dinner." She got out the cereals, I got out the bowls—the biggest ones I could find. It was our entire dinner after all. She promptly replaced hers with a much smaller bowl and a regular spoon instead of the big soup spoon I selected. Feeling guilty I did the same.

Her diet secret was smaller dishes and smaller utensils. She said when she changed from oversized dinner plates to salad plates and from pasta bowls to small soup bowls her weight scaled down as well.

The Food Spy

When I feel a little out of control with cravings, I spy on others. If I'm tempted to fill my grocery basket with junk foods because I'm hungry, I look around at the baskets of other shoppers. Without even looking at the shopper you can tell if they are in shape. The larger the person, the more junk food in their basket. The slimmer the shopper, the more fresh and healthy food they're buying.

At the grocery prepared-food counters, which have become lifesavers for today's busy women, watch who buys what. It will not be a slim person helping themselves to the saucy ribs and potato salad but the one with the sliced turkey breast and fresh fruit salad most likely will be. Don't feel deprived, feel empowered.

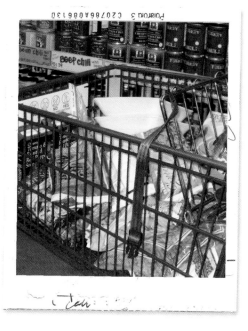

Cocktails

My New York literary friend introduced me to the cosmopolitan cocktail on one of my working visits. Not only was it pretty, it was delicious and dissipated the stress of the day. Have a few cosmos a few times too many and you'll need to move the button on your pants. Alcoholic beverages are tasty, social, and soothing, but high in calories.

Do you have to become a teetotaler? No, but you must pick your times. A special dinner, a special drink, fine. You can't have it all. Actually you can if you give equal consideration to your weight and food. Really, isn't a slim hipline as good as a chardonnay? Isn't a smaller waistline as fulfilling as a lemon drop martini?

The greener the inside of the basket, the healthier. What color is yours?

Coffee Breaks

Look in my wallet and you will see my hole-punched Coffee Bean card. Only after a month of daily coffeehouse visits did I realize that I was gaining weight. I was doing the same exercise routine and eating the same moderate diet. The only difference was my coffee breaks. I had never thought to find out the caloric and fat content because I ordered nonfat, decaffeinated drinks, of course without the whip cream.

On my next visit I asked about the ingredients and they gave me a printed sheet that almost knocked the wind out of me. My coffees were indeed nonfat, but those delicious flavorings—in that tiny scoop or pump hid fattening little calories. I had to alter my routine. Do I want to pull my car over as I drive by a Coffee Bean? You betcha, but I also want to fit in my clothes. It's all about what you want more.

Eating Out

One of the hardest things about healthy eating is eating out. Somehow in our own homes we can control our eating better, or so we think we can. What happens when we walk through the doorway of a restaurant or a friend's home? Most of our discipline stays outside. We need to move it inside.

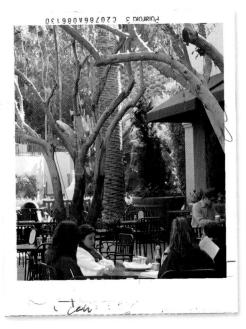

Here are a few things that work for me when I eat out:

- Stay away from buffets. Really, who has that kind of discipline?
- Order à la carte.
- Have the plates removed as soon as you finish eating.
- Don't even let them set down the breadbasket and butter dish. We are only human after all.
- Have a nonfat, decaf cappuccino for your dessert and sip it slowly.
- Don't arrive starved. I always eat a healthy little something before I walk out the door. It goes against the grain of everything my mother told me, but now I *want* to ruin my dinner just a bit.

FAST FOOD

You really have to stay out of fast-food restaurants. You just do. I call them fat-food restaurants. Yes, they do save you time and many think money, but I disagree. Don't believe those campaigns about the new fast-food "diet sandwiches" because most often they hide some yummy, caloric sauce between the lettuce and the tomato to make it taste better.

Answers?

Where do you go to get the information you need to make healthful food choices? This magazine says one thing, another says something else. I have had many doctors taking nutrition classes alongside me and it frightens me to realize they know so little. Television spokespersons are sometimes less than expert. Anyone who looks good enough and has a gift of gab can become a television "expert." Some are indeed what the title implies, but how do you tell the difference? Just as in everything else, the bottom line is what works for you.

Diet Pills

When I was in college the drug of choice for women was diet pills. Everyone was looking for the underground supply, the secret to thinness. Today there are hundreds of brands of over-the-counter diet pills that promise miracles. If they really worked there would be no best-selling diet books. If they worked, we would all be lining up to buy them. The stores couldn't control the mobs. You think a Macy's sale is madness?

GROWN-UP GIRL'S DIETS RULE:

Diets don't work. Retrain you brain to eat sensibly and healthy.
It's all about your choices. Choose yourself.

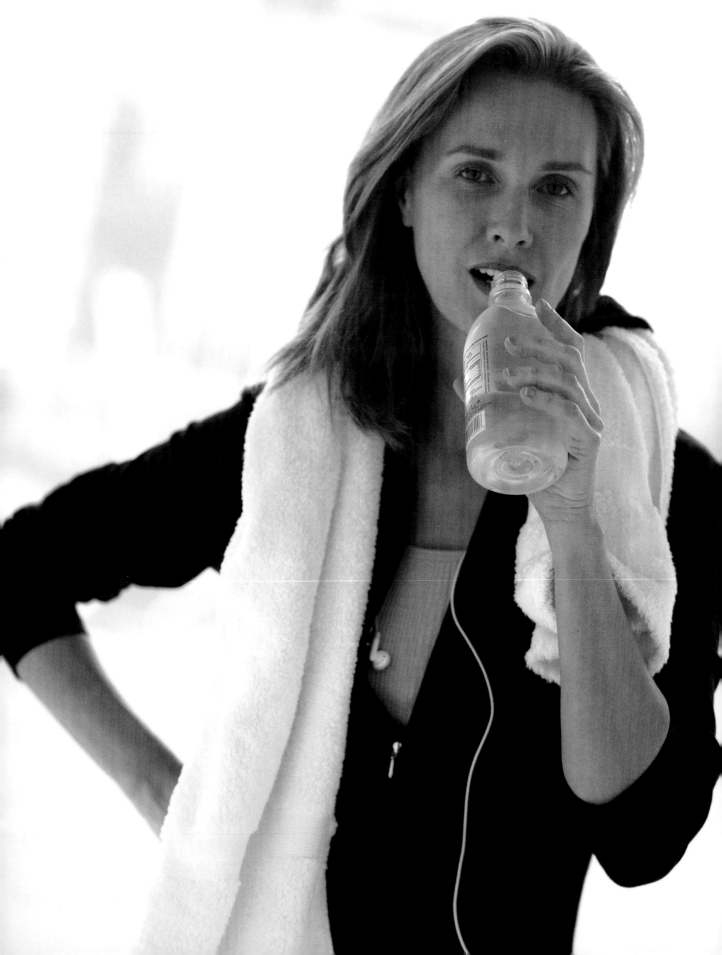

CHAPTER ELEVEN

Exercise

There isn't a doctor or professional alive that will tell you not to exercise if you can move any part of your body. We are meant to move, and the more grown up we are, the more we need the movement.

Attitude

As our bodies adjust to growing up, so must our activity level. While the ups and downs of raising children and/or careers might have been enough to keep our weight under control during our thirties, this is usually not enough as we pass forty. We have to shake up our routines, readjust, and find what works now. It's so very simple. Movement equals weight loss. The faster the movement, the bigger the loss. You must burn more calories than you take in. Why do we make it so complicated? How you pay the price is up to you, as long as you pay.

The Payment Plan

I TiVo my favorite television shows and view them only on the treadmill or the bicycle. I don't allow myself to watch them any other place. I can hardly wait to get to my gym when I have a new episode of *Without a Trace*. A one-hour drama equals my cardiovascular workout. A half-hour sitcom completes my weight-bearing training.

Nobody says things like Oprah. She cuts to the chase. She says it the way we always wish we could. On the topic of exercise she says quite simply, "Just get moving."

On the Road

Upon arriving in the Big Apple from California about nine one evening and checking into my hotel, I indulged in a minibar extravaganza. After the munching came the guilt. The gym was closed, so I started jogging in place. I added a few jumping jacks here and there, moved around the bed and into the bathroom and kept moving. Luckily *Desperate Housewives* was on, so I kept going, through the commercials and right up to the end. One hour of nonstop movement. I call it my "no-excuse" workout.

Private Trainers

I don't like private trainers on a regular basis. I like to do my own thing. That is a personal preference. I feel you need a trainer to get you going and to tweak you every once in a while.

My experience at gyms has been that many people hire private trainers just to chat. The conversations I overhear belong in a therapist's office or over coffee with a good friend. If you hire a trainer, make sure it's your body that's moving, not your mouth.

Shake It Up

Vary your exercise routine. If you normally exercise inside, go outside. If you go to the gym, try a studio class. Give yourself a new setting. There are so many types of work-outs and so many different places to do them, take advantage and keep your exercise life as interesting as the rest of your life. This is one relationship where monogamy is not important. Play the field.

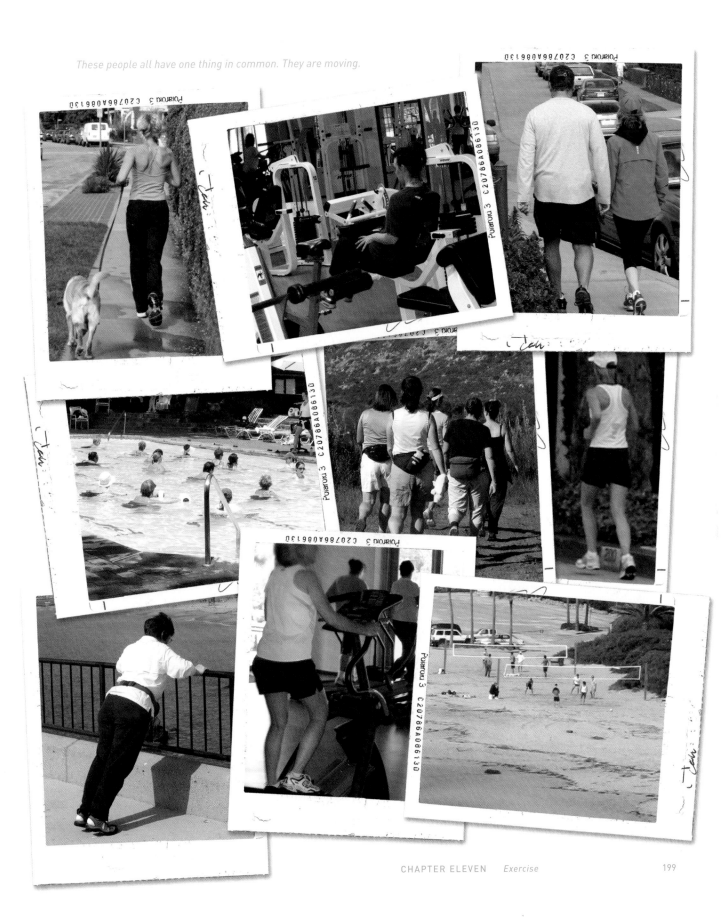

These people all have one thing in common. They are moving.

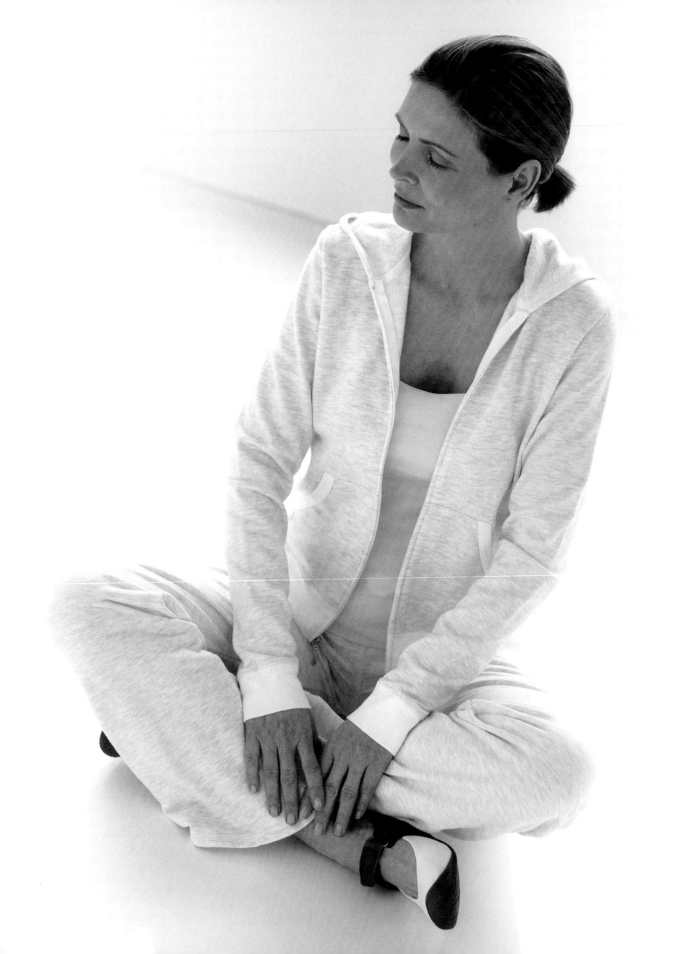

CHAPTER TWELVE

Health

The saying "if you have your health you have everything" doesn't impress anyone under thirty. Health is usually not an issue for them. Only when you or someone near you loses their health do you understand the reality of this statement.

Control Freaks

When it comes to your health care, you want to be known as a control freak. If you do not take charge of your own health care you can be in serious trouble. The very best doctors, at the top-notch hospitals, do not always have the time to watch over your health the way you do. They are trying to care for many patients, you have only one. I like the odds of one to one far better than one hundred to one.

Today health care is a blending of the medical world with the holistic world. Yet, these worlds continue to rival each other. Medical doctors are often offended that you are also listening to a homeopathic doctor. Alternative doctors often feel that medical treatments are too toxic. The enduring question is how to blend tradition with uncharted territories. You cannot be intimidated. You have to be the one in charge. You must make the decisions based on all the information you can gather. It's your life, your health, and your peace of mind. Only once you have explored all the possibilities can you decide what is right for you.

GROWN-UP GIRL'S HEALTH RULE:
Don't talk about health all the time. Fill your time with talk about life.

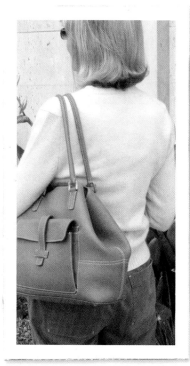

Six months with this oversized stylish purse and I bet she will be tilting to one side.

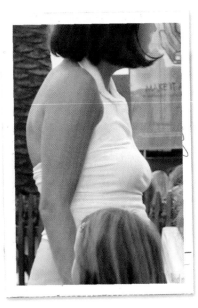

It doesn't matter what you're wearing if your posture is bad.

Nonfunctioning Tables

I have put a ban on any body function talk at dinner tables. I had to. Everyone wants to compare ailments and cholesterol numbers. It's not that I don't care, it's that there are far more interesting things to discuss while dining. We all know men get prostate problems. We live with menstrual issues. We just don't need to share them at social functions. Save them for intimate phone calls if you must, but please save them.

I find the most interesting people never talk about health. They don't focus on the past. They live in the present. They are interested in you: who you are, what you do, and what you like. They discuss current things with you, not at you. They listen. You never know their cholesterol numbers. Who could even remember?

The Upright Back

When we turn forty, talk starts to turn to osteoporosis. *Calcium* becomes a fundamental word in our vocabularies and an essential item in our medicine chests. Yet, to our own detriment, we continue to carry heavy purses, hunch over our computers, and talk with the phone between our shoulder and ear as we multitask. Old habits are hard to break.

Good posture is crucial to our maintenance. Hope Gillerman is a certified instructor of the Alexander Technique in New York City, where she works daily teaching women balance and correct posture. Here is her advice:

- Stretch. Stretch. Stretch.
- Stop doing crunches, they collapse you.
- Train your muscles to do what you want them to do, standing up to lengthen your spine.
- Do reverse crunches. First, lie on your back, arms at sides, knees bent, and feet on floor by hips. Pull your belly button back toward the floor, and flatten your back. Second, still on your back, all at once lift your legs and hips up off the floor. Repeat ten times. Keep your upper back on the floor.

- Use a wall, fridge, anything straight to practice how the abdominal muscles lift you up. With your back to the wall, place heels about 4 inches from the wall and hips against the wall. Just the tips of the shoulder blades touch the wall, not your head. Bend knees slightly. Put your hands on your lower abdomen, between the pubic bone and the belly button. Pull your hands back toward the wall, lifting up as you go, like spreading out a sheet. This should bring you closer to the wall. This is the posture you want all the time.

- Work on balance by standing on one leg, lifting the abdominals up and holding the position as long as possible. Do this while talking on the phone so you will breathe properly. The better our balance, the better our posture. This is the posture you want all the time, lower back lengthened, abdominals lifting.

- Check your posture in mirrors.

- In the case of bags, size doesn't matter. It's what you put inside them that create the problems.

- Carry things symmetrically with your body. Hug items to your chest, not balanced on your hip.

- Wedge shoes throw your body out of balance. Vary your heel heights.

- At your computer have a chair that has a flat back or lumbar support. Don't arch your back as you work. Keyboards need to be at the level where our shoulders are not rounded, and close enough so our backs are not hunched.

- Try Pilates, stretch classes, yoga, swimming, or any exercise that stretches your body.

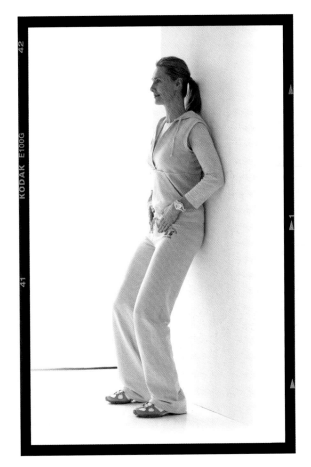

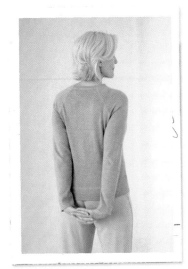

Posture Exercise

For the last four years I have made a yearly visit to Rancho La Puerta in Mexico. Think Canyon Ranch on a budget. It is one of my absolute favorite vacations. I love to observe the people the day they enter the ranch and then a week later as they leave. I swear they look taller. In reality they stand taller because their bodies are stretched and relaxed. One of my favorite exercises from the ranch is a very simple posture adjuster:

- Stand still with your feet apart.
- Clasp your hands behind your back, elbows straight.
- Pull your shoulders down, keeping your hands clasped.
- Hold for at least one minute.

Go Figure

We have grown up with the myth "You can never be too rich or too thin." The thin part of this myth desperately needs changing. Reed-thin on a twenty-year-old is model material. That same thinness on a forty, fifty, or sixty-year-old is aging. For older, mature models, or "classic," as the modeling agencies describe them, thin becomes gaunt, and progresses to wrinkled. Opt for a few extra pounds rather than a few less.

For us the emphasis needs to change from thin to fit. Fit is healthy. It means you exercise and eat right. Whatever your size, strive for form. Full-figure models look incredible in their size sixteens and eighteens simply because they are athletic. They understand the importance of working out and keeping their extra size firm.

GROWN-UP GIRL'S WEIGHT RULE:

Change the word *thin* to the word *fit* in your conversations and your life.

The Pill Box

Our pill box changes as we get older. Bone density is not in the vocabulary of the young. For the woman approaching menopause or in menopause it is a major factor. As our age increases our bone density has a tendency to decrease.

Today it's all about prevention. A good diet strong in calcium-enriched foods is the beginning. A daily multivitamin or stress tab is important if your eating habits are compromised. Add on a lot of bone density exercises and you're in the prevention mode.

The preeminent news is that you cannot only maintain your bone density, with today's medications you can actually increase it.

Dr. Edward Liu's busy OB/GYN practice consists of women of all ages. He delivered many babies for the women he now treats for aging issues. There is help in the world of osteoporosis if you check your bone density early. To keep bones from getting brittle, there are several avenues to pursue.

Over-the-counter products:

- Take 1500 to 2000 milligrams of calcium a day. Vitamin D helps absorption. Choose from several forms:
    - Calcium tablets—strength varies; check the label.
    - Viactive—chewy candy with 500 milligrams of calcium in every cube.
    - Tums or extra-strength Rolaids—see the label for calcium level.

Prescription drugs:

- Fosamax, Actonel, and Boniva—made from bisphosphonates which inhibit bone resorption.
- Evista—a SERM (selective estrogen receptor modulator) which mimics the benefit of estrogen on bones and cholesterol without the adverse risks of hormone-related cancers.
- Miacalcin—a nasal spray derived from calcitonin produced by the thyroid gland which prevents bone resorption.

To bring back bone density:

- Forteo—a new medication given in daily shots over a restricted period of time. Derived from parathyroid hormone.
- HRT—hormone replacement therapy.

The big question for women over forty is whether to use estrogens. A few years ago a study that was supposed to run seven years was stopped abruptly after three because they said it caused breast cancer and everyone ran scared. Of course the media agitated the situation with their sensational hype. Little by little the study got picked apart and once again doctors and patients came to believe that hormones wouldn't cause breast cancer. The media didn't make such a big deal out of *these* findings.

Dr. Edward Liu, leading obstetrician/gynecologist at Cedars-Sinai in Los Angeles says, "estrogens aren't totally out of the question in selected patients." Estrogens treat memory loss, bone density, heart disease, cholesterol, skin elasticity, and libido. There are other drugs on the market that you can take for bones, heart, and cholesterol that don't cause cancer. Unfortunately, there are very few replacements for estrogen when it comes to loss of memory, skin elasticity, and sex drive. Estrogens are antiaging drugs. Women have the choice, it's up to them to make the decision. It's not a doctor's decision, it's a conversation between a woman and her doctor. Only a woman can make the final decision on estrogens. Dr. Liu said one of his patients came to him wanting to take estrogen again after watching her mother suffer from Alzheimer's disease. She said she would rather take her chances with breast cancer. How can anyone dispute her choice?

Hormone Replacement

Dr. Edward Liu's suggestions on hormone replacement therapy:

- First try over-the-counter products such as Estroven, Promensil, Remifemin, and Healthy Woman Soy-Menopause Pill. They may be enough for your body. All of these are branded products. Generic soy and black cohosh will work, too.
- If nonprescription remedies are not enough, go to the lowest level of estrogens. The solutions should match your symptoms.
- Be a minimalist in terms of how much medication you need to treat your symptoms.
- All hormone therapy must be customized by the doctor for the patient.
- Have mammograms, pap smears, and yearly physicals on schedule.
- Take into consideration your family's health history. Chances are you will inherit some of their problems. Good news is you have insight and can get a head start on prevention treatment.

S-E-X

Most men, regardless of age, are interested, very interested, in sex. Why else do they divorce and marry much younger women? Three letters, S-E-X. Men at every age love sex. They love to feel sexy, they love to be sexy, they love a sexy mate. So why do they hang out in front of the television set, clicking between sports and news, and perhaps the erotic channels when their mates are fast asleep?

I am not a sex therapist, I am a woman in a second marriage; a healthy, sexy, second marriage. Here are some of my tips:

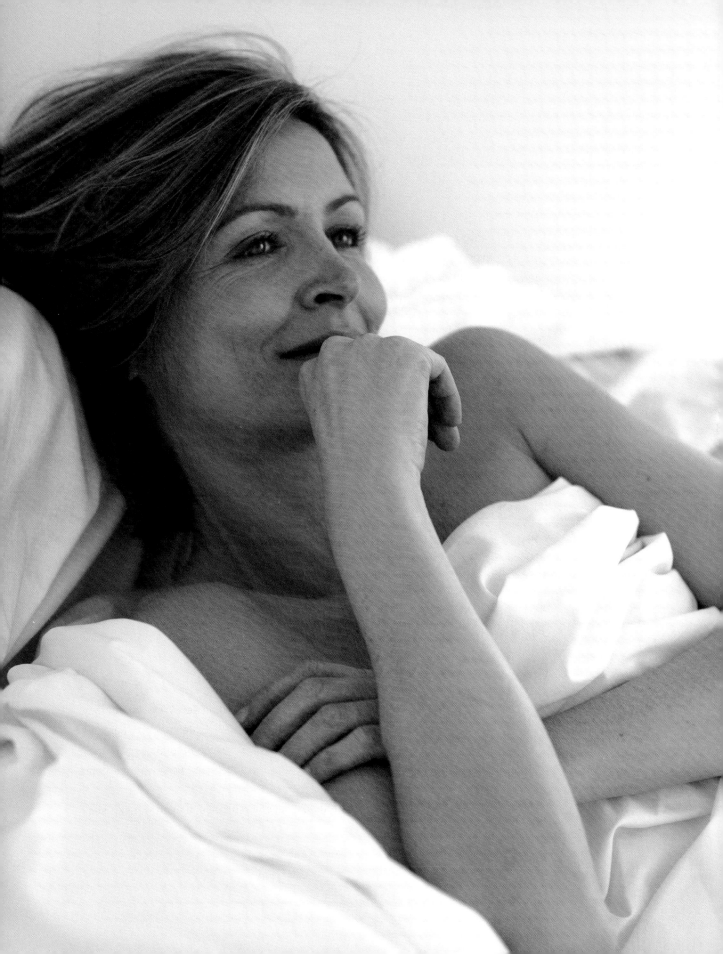

- If you work in the boardroom, don't take it into the bedroom. You might be the head of a company during the day, but the briefcase mode should stay behind when you come home.
- Think about what turned on your man when you were first together. Then stop thinking and do it.

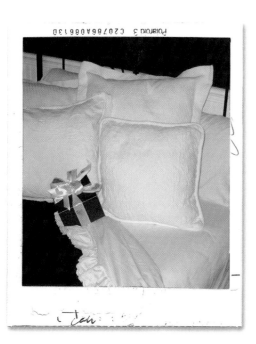

- Be sexy. Don't save sex for when you get in bed. Surprise your mate when he least expects it. Surprise him in different areas of the house. Surprise him at different times of the day. Just don't surprise him when his favorite team is playing. It will only hurt your ego.
- Send him little notes. Hide them in his medicine chest, in his wallet, or on the back of the TV clicker.
- Make surprise dates. Plan an outing just for the two of you. Not everything has to be done with friends.
- Make your bedroom romantic with music, candles, and nice linens. Don't save the good stuff for the guests.
- Plan a romantic getaway weekend. Buy something new to sleep in. Try a new perfume.
- Buy him something. I hide presents inside the bed, on his side. He loves it.
- Keep yourself vibrant. Hopefully it will influence him to do the same.
- Tell him you love him. Who ever hears it enough?

I don't believe that *all* the responsibility falls on women. But I do feel that women, being the smarter sex, especially when it comes to affairs of the heart (or the bedroom) need to be the ones to take the initiative. Couples need to think of marriage as an extension of the love affair. How did they dress and act during the courting days? We shouldn't get too comfortable or take each other for granted. Maintaining your appearance is one of the nicest gifts you can give each other. Letting yourself go is not fair and it's not smart, for either of you. It doesn't mean you both sit around in elaborate clothing, it means you both take the time to look nice for each other.

Dr. Edward Liu's Libido Tips

Viagra has changed the sex lives of mature men. All of a sudden a man has his young erection back, but his mate might not have her once-young vagina. How do we find a balance? Some women have tried Viagra and found that while it increases their sexual response, it does nothing for their head. We all know that for most of us sex is as much about the head as it is about the vagina.

Your doctor and a compounding pharmacist can work together to make the hormones in the form you want to use: mouth, skin, or vagina. The patient has to decide what her needs are and what she is willing to do for results.

- Oral medications may not be enough to treat the vaginal symptoms. Topical, local products may be necessary.
- A compounding pharmacy can supply:
  - *A little jelly and a little testosterone for a vaginal lubricating cream*
  - *A few drops of diluted testosterone to be placed under the tongue*
  - *The testosterone pills that men put under their gums can be used (off-brand and off-label) by some women. They are halved or quartered and placed inside the vagina. Instant libido!*
  - *All of these treatments, unlike Viagra for men, must be used on a regular basis.*
  - *Estrogen creams, patches, and vaginal rings are other ways to replace hormones in your body.*

Lube Jobs

Grown-up girls sometime need lubrication. Topical creams and gels work but can be messy. The internal Estring O ring sounded over the top when my doctor first told me about it, but once I got used to the idea I found it is a major improvement over all the other products.

There are many lubricants on the drugstore shelf. Try something light and non-greasy. Try the ones that heat up with your touch. Now, we're talking hot! It needs to be applied to the man so make it part of your foreplay. This is one area where women still don't talk to each other and are even shy to ask their doctors. Why should they be? When I was twenty I didn't think anyone over fifty had sex. Now I know the truth.

The sex lives of grown-up men and women are changing radically because of the advancement in medications. Don't rule them out. Half the fun is in the testing.

GROWN-UP GIRL'S SEX TALK RULE:
Don't talk about your sex life—live it.

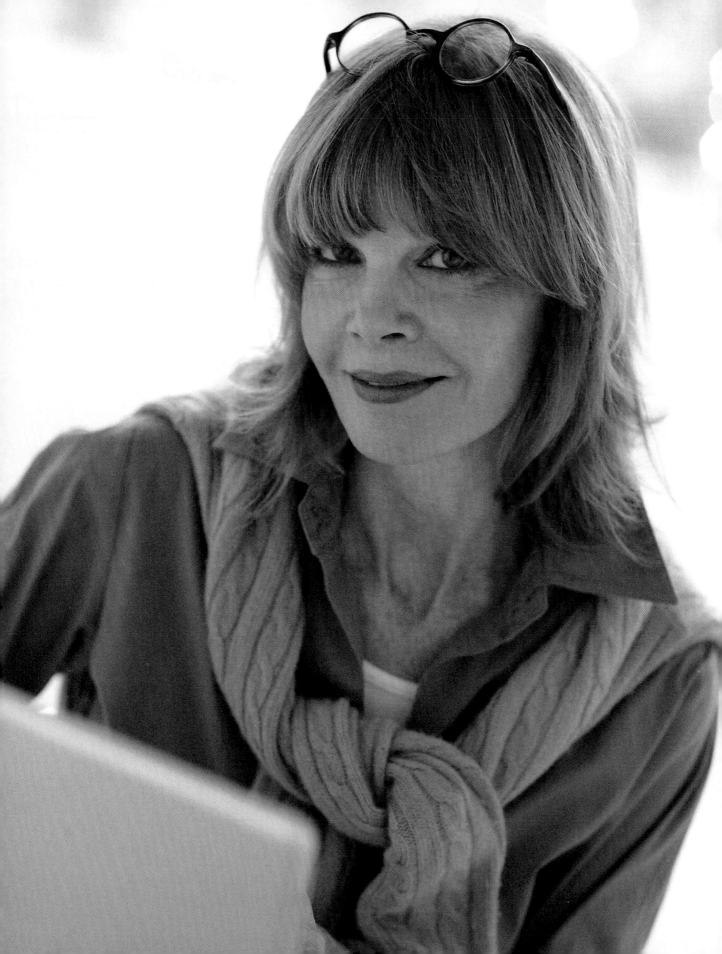

CHAPTER THIRTEEN

Life as a Grown-Up Girl

My Role Model

I truly believe you can be an ageless woman. I am fortunate because I have a good role model. All of us who love her call her Grandma Z. This year she will celebrate a birthday somewhere in the nineties. I don't know exactly which one because it's really not important to Grandma Z or to me.

She is a grown-up girl who has always lived her life to its fullest. Where she once traveled around the world, she now makes an event of a trip to the bookstore searching for a delicious novel. A lunch at one of her favorite local spots now replaces a business dinner party.

She challenges her mind with weekly computer lessons. She challenges her friends with interesting topics of conversation. She is always redecorating a room in her home or planting a new area in her lovely garden. She isn't scaling down her life; she is always trying to expand it.

Grandma Z doesn't want to focus on health, she wants to focus on you. She doesn't dwell on her aches and pains, she tries to outlive them. Her daily goal is to go out and experience life. She doesn't live in the past, she lives in the present and talks about the future. She is not waiting to die, she is striving to live.

When I am with her I don't realize the difference of years between our ages. They are not important. What is important is that she is interesting and interested. There's a sparkle about my friend. A twinkle in her eyes that lets you know there is indeed a good quality of life at any age. She has that sparkle and twinkle because she continually works at creating them. She keeps her life full, stimulating, and progressive. She does not give up or give in. She keeps moving forward.

My goal in life is to emulate Grandma Z. She sets the bar high, but the rewards are even higher. In my mind, she sets a standard for which all grown-up girls should strive.

The Journey

This may be the end of our book journey together, but it's only the beginning of your amazing life after forty. You have the choice to be ageless. Only *you* can make the changes to initiate this choice.

Maya Angelou said, "The 50s are everything you've been meaning to be." But for some of you growing up starts in the forties or it sneaks up on you in the sixties. It really doesn't matter at what age you move into the grown-up world, it only matters how you do it. It's important that you become everything you've been meaning to be. Keep laughing with your friends and family; continue to challenge your mind. Always appreciate the miracle of your body and treat yourself with the utmost respect. Never stop reminiscing over old memories as you continue to make new ones. Take a minute every single day to appreciate the gifts of life. All that matters is that you continue on the roller coaster of life for as long as possible, always focusing on the highs.

MY GROWN-UP GIRL'S RULE FOR LIFE:
"SAVOR IT!"

Acknowledgments

I have lived *The Grown-Up Girl's Guide to Style* for quite a few years now and have toyed with the idea of sharing it. But when I thought about revealing all my secrets, I moved on to something else. Finally, with the help of many important people in my life, I am able to "bare all" on paper.

Every writer needs mentors, and I have two of the best.

Phyllis Melhado has continuously encouraged my writing. I turn to her for professional advice, support, and friendship and she is always there.

Julia Serebrinsky came to me through business but quickly became a treasured friend. Her enthusiasm and support helped me put my ideas on paper.

Thanks to my agent Carol Mann for loving the *Grown-Up Girls* from the very beginning.

From the conception of this idea I wanted Judith Regan to publish this book because she has proven that she has her pulse on the reading taste of America. Special applause to Cassie, Richard, and Maureen for making it happen.

Thanks to my photographer Michael Donnelly, he is a true artist and visionary; to my stylist Diana Sheppard, one of the most tasteful women I know; and to Steve Hanselman for his brilliant business mind and positive direction.

For generous help with my proposal, thank you Steve Miller for printing; and Chris Jacquemin, Ave Butenski, The Simmons Research Group, and Cotton Inc. for research.

Last, but forever first in my life, I thank my incredible husband, Shelly Schwab, for his love and encouragement. Life with him is this grown-up girl's dream come true.